"Combining scientific data and ancient wisdom,
this skillfully written book makes a compelling case. . .
If you eat, you should read this book."

—Chade-Meng Tan, bestselling author of *Search Inside Yourself*

"Scientists have known for years that time-restricted
diets protect against obesity and other metabolic diseases.
Buddha's Diet brings these findings to the world."

—Dr. Satchidananda Panda, Salk Institute for Biological
Sciences, one of the world's leading experts on time-restricted diets

buddha's diet

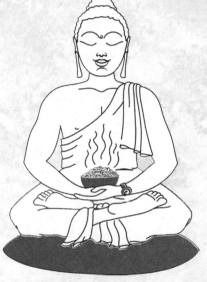

the ancient art of losing weight without losing your mind

TARA COTTRELL AND DAN ZIGMOND

Running Press

PHILADELPHIA · LONDON

Published by Running Press,
An imprint of Perseus Books, a Division of PBG Publishing, LLC,
A subsidiary of Hachette Book Group

ISBN 978-0-7624-6046-5
Library of Congress Control Number: 2016941457

E-book ISBN 978-0-7624-6047-2

9 8 7 6 5 4 3 2 1
Digit on the right indicates the number of this printing

Cover design by Sarah Pierson
Interior design by Amanda Richmond
Edited by Jennifer Kasius
Typography: Garamond, Blog Script, and Brandon.

Running Press Book Publishers
2300 Chestnut Street
Philadelphia, PA 19103-4371

Visit us on the web!
www.runningpress.com

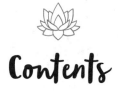

Contents

The pudgy guy in Chinese restaurants is not Buddha—Buddha was actually in pretty good shape. He tried dieting once and didn't like it any more than you do. But he eventually developed some basic rules for eating that still make sense today.

PART 1: INSIGHTS

Some of the latest research on obesity has confirmed Buddha's original teaching about eating: *When* we eat is as important as *what* we eat. We weren't designed to eat at all hours of the day. Now we know why.

Buddha taught that we should take nothing on faith. So what does the evidence say about why we get fat? And why is it so hard to get thin again? The answer, and the surprising solution, is part of why Buddha's Diet works.

PART 4: PERFECTIONS

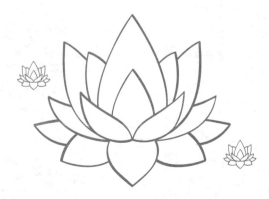

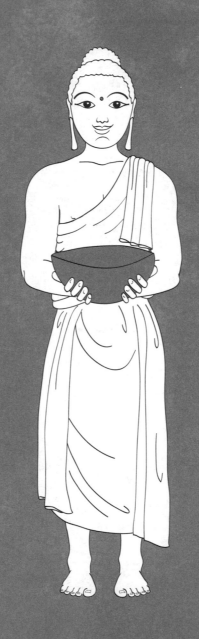

INTRODUCTION

Buddha Was Thin

THERE'S A LOT YOU DON'T KNOW ABOUT BUDDHA.

To start with, Buddha was thin. The pudgy statues you see smiling at you at Chinese restaurants and yoga studios aren't actually Buddha—or not *the* Buddha anyway, not the one who lived in ancient India and meditated a lot and ultimately began teaching what we now call Buddhism. That chubby guy is a fabled monk who wandered the Chinese countryside at least a thousand years later, performing minor magic and predicting the future. Over the years he became a folk hero and a symbol of happiness and good fortune. He's especially popular in Japan these days, where they call him Hotei (pronounced *hoe-tay*) and see him as a jolly old man—a little like Santa Claus, but handing out luck instead of toys.

Hotei muddied the waters a bit by composing a poem on his deathbed suggesting he might have been the reincarnation of some *other* Buddha. But he was certainly not the original Buddha. Statues and paintings of the *real* Buddha typically show him as lean and trim—even in his younger years as a pampered prince. (More on that in a minute.) By all accounts he was a pretty good-looking guy. Buddha was many things over the course of his life, but he was never fat.

In fact, you'll sometimes see images of the Buddha looking downright skeletal. Those depict the years when Buddha was on a diet. That's right—Buddha tried dieting, too. And it worked—sort of. They say he lost so much weight that his ribs "jutted out as gaunt as the crazy rafters of an old roofless barn"[1] and if you touched his stomach you could feel his spine.[2] In other words, he got *thin* thin.

Buddha wasn't dieting to look good in a swimsuit. He wasn't even technically the Buddha yet. He was just a normal guy a little confused about life. Back then, there was already a long tradition in India of trying to liberate the mind through conquering the body. Modern yoga has its roots in these ascetic practices, which involved not just stretching your body into proscribed poses and postures, but sleeping on a bed of nails, beating yourself with branches, holding your breath for minutes on end, and fasting for days, weeks, even months at a time. That's what Buddha was trying.

To understand how he got to that point, you need to know a bit more about his life story. Buddha was born into a royal family in India about twenty-five hundred years ago. They gave him the hopeful name of Siddhartha, which means roughly "the one who achieves his goals."[3] There were various miracles around his birth, and a local soothsayer foretold that Siddhartha would grow up to be either a powerful ruler or a great sage. This was no contest for his father and mother—being royals themselves, they wanted him to go the ruler route. They became the original helicopter parents and did everything they could to shelter him from the slightest pain or discomfort, trying to steer him firmly toward the secular. They banned anything that might lead him down the spiritual path, even posting guards at the gates to keep all unhappy people away. They filled his life with every luxury imaginable.

Like most attempts to shelter our kids, this worked for a while—and then it didn't. Siddhartha had a nagging feeling that there was more to life than fun and games. One day he convinced his servant to help him sneak out of the palace grounds. As he rode his horse through the local village, he had his first encounters with real human suffering. He saw sickness, old age, and death. And all of a sudden, he realized he couldn't continue his life in his parents' artificial Shangri-La and vowed to make a change. He saw one of those wandering ascetics crisscrossing India, and decided to give that life a try.

So that's how Siddhartha ended up on a crazy diet and looking much like a corpse. He probably didn't like dieting any more than you do. And worse, it didn't *really* work. He lost weight, of course—anyone can lose weight temporarily if they completely stop eating—but it didn't bring him any closer to enlightenment. It certainly didn't point him toward the end of suffering. It only made him suffer *more*.

Siddhartha had starved himself nearly to death by the time he figured out he had to stop. Denying his body even the most basic sustenance wasn't any better than his parents' approach of wallowing in every possible pleasure. And he saw that if he continued any longer, his life would simply end. He would die right there, no better off, no wiser than when he left home.

Luckily, at that exact moment, a young girl walked by and saw him sitting there pathetically, nearly on his last breath. She felt sorry for him and offered him some milk. He accepted it gratefully, and the milk saved his life and gave him enough strength to continue his meditations. That's when he realized that food was not an enemy to be resisted. Food was essential to sustain his body, and his body was essential to living a meaningful life. There had to be a middle ground between torturing himself like the ascetics and indulging his every whim like his parents.

With that realization, Siddhartha experienced enlightenment. He became the Buddha—which literally means the "awakened one." It was as if he had been asleep all his life, alternating between sweet dreams and horrible nightmares, and then finally he woke up.

Buddha went on to become a great teacher, just as the soothsayer predicted, traveling around what is now India and Nepal expounding on his "middle way." After his death, these teachings spread farther, eventually covering nearly all of Asia. In the twentieth century, they reached Europe, Africa, and the Americas, too.

The Buddha taught *a lot*. The oldest collections of his lectures run about 20,000 pages. Seriously. The Chinese versions—which add some lectures they say were discovered later—are a whopping 80,000 pages. To put that in perspective, the Bible has around 1,000 pages. And the Bible is the work of several teachers—Moses, the Prophets, the Apostles, Saint Paul, etc. So Buddha's teachings would fill somewhere between 20 and 80 whole Bibles, depending on whom you ask, all composed by one guy.

Buddha lectured on almost every topic you can imagine, but once he decided it was okay to eat now and then, he didn't seem to think that much about food. He mentions it only a few times in all those thousands and thousands of pages.

And honestly, you shouldn't think too much about food, either. But you probably do.

This book looks at Buddha's middle way as it applies to eating. We call it Buddha's Diet. It isn't complicated or expensive. You don't need to join a club or buy special meals or juices. There aren't obscure ingredients to eat every day or to banish from your kitchen altogether. You just need to follow a few guidelines that Buddha worked out. These will help you lose weight and feel better and eventually stop thinking about food much at all.

But why should you care what some Indian guy said about dieting over two thousand years ago? Haven't we learned a lot about food and nutrition since then?

You'd be surprised.

A lot of what we thought we learned has turned out not to be true. Cholesterol was bad, and then it wasn't. We substituted sugar for fat, then found out that was the wrong way around. Not everyone can agree if meat is healthy or not, or if soy is better or worse. Countless fad diets have come and gone. And through it all, we're still getting fatter and fatter, and less and less healthy.

Luckily we're finally starting to see some good science on eating and obesity. And believe it or not, many of the best recent results echo Buddha's original teachings. The former prince was on to something.

Buddha's teachings were all about moderation. A lot of us are stuck in the same extremes Buddha rejected—eating everything that's not nailed down one month, then starving ourselves on some crazy diet the next. And it doesn't work. We end up overweight and unhappy, wasting time fighting with food when we should be living our lives. Buddha's Diet can help you change that.

You'll lose weight without losing your mind.

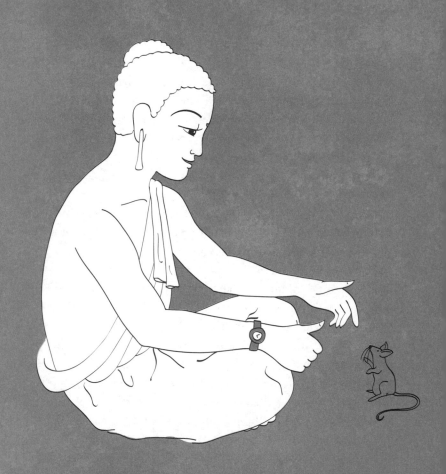

PART 1

INSIGHTS

CHAPTER 1

Of Mice and Monks

PEOPLE HAVE BEEN TELLING EACH OTHER WHAT TO EAT for thousands of years. Most of the major religions around the world include some sort of dietary restrictions. Islam prohibits pork. Orthodox Jews refrain from mixing milk and meat. Catholics avoid certain foods during Lent. Some devout Hindus don't just eschew eating animals, but also shy away from certain root vegetables because harvesting them kills the plant.

Back when Buddha laid down rules for his followers, he didn't follow this pattern. In the West we often assume that Buddhists are vegetarians—and certainly some of them are—but that's not generally the case. Nothing in the original Buddhist scriptures prohibits eating meat, and there are many ancient stories of the Buddha and his first disciples eating all kinds of food.[1] Some people are surprised to learn that even His Holiness the Dalai Lama eats meat—and grew up eating almost nothing else, since very few plants grow well in the harsh altitudes of Tibet. To this day in most of Asia, Buddhist vegetarians are the exception, not the rule.

In fact, although he gave incredibly detailed instructions on things like where his monks could sleep and what they could wear, the Buddha said very little about what his followers could or couldn't eat. On the contrary, tradition stated that monks should eat whatever was offered to them. In much of Southeast Asia, saffron-robed monks can still be seen making their alms rounds every morning, and then eating whatever their generous neighbors put in their begging bowls.

The one strict gastronomic rule the Buddha prescribed was that monks should avoid what he called "untimely eating." Specifically, they should eat only between dawn and noon.[2] Afternoon and evening eating was strictly prohibited. The Buddha didn't care too much *what* monks ate, but he cared a lot *when* they ate it.

This may sound like an odd and nitpicky restriction, but Buddha clearly meant it seriously. When he later boiled down the 227 rules he had made for monks into a sort of top-ten list for novices in training, the first few were the ones you might expect—rules like no killing and no stealing. But his funny dietary restriction also made the cut.[3] When he whittled them down to eight rules that laypeople could observe if they wanted to get more serious about Buddhism, he included that they "should not eat at night or at an improper time."[4]

The Buddha gave a few different explanations for this seeming obsession with meal schedules. But one of his clearest was this:

> Monks, I do not eat in the evening. Because I avoid eating in the evening, I am in good health, light, energetic, and live comfortably. You, too, monks, avoid eating in the evening, and you will have good health.[5]

Fast-forward to 2014, when Dr. Satchidananda Panda and his team of researchers at the prestigious Salk Institute for Biological Sciences in California published a fascinating study on obesity in mice.[6] They took one group of mice and instead of their normal chow, they offered them a diet of high-fat, high-calorie foods, and let them eat as much as they wanted. The results would surprise no one: the mice got fat.

Then they took another group of mice and offered them exactly the same seemingly unhealthy diet, but this time they only let the mice eat for nine to twelve hours each day. During the rest of the day and night, the mice got only water. In other words, these mice had the same all-you-can-eat buffet of tasty, fattening treats for most of their waking hours. The one rule was that they could only stuff themselves during *some* of their waking hours.

The scientists called this "time-restricted feeding," and we'll go into a lot more detail about the study in the chapter "Eating Like a Mouse." But for now, suffice it to say that this time, the results *were* a surprise: *none of these mice got fat.* Something about matching their eating to their natural circadian rhythms seemed to protect the mice against all that otherwise fattening food. It didn't matter if they loaded up with sugars and fats. It didn't seem to matter *what* the mice ate, or even how much of it—only *when* they ate it.

Somehow Buddha and the biologists had come to roughly the same conclusion.

While much of the world still worries about starvation and malnutrition, here in the United States and other wealthy countries, obesity is a far greater concern. In many ways, this is an achievement. Most of us no longer fear wasting away after a bad drought or poor crop—fears that plagued humanity for most of history and still do in too many other places. Instead we live like the happy but unfortunate mice in that first experiment, surrounded by cheap, delicious food that we consume whenever we want.

Yet this blessing has become a curse. The health risks of obesity have become well known, but a few bear repeating: heart disease, high blood pressure, diabetes.[7] Millions of Americans die from these weight-related diseases every year. Despite advances in medical care, by one estimate serious obesity still robs an average woman of *seven years* of life when all the health risks are added together.[8] We are literally eating ourselves to death.

As if that wasn't enough, there are real financial costs, too. Researchers at George Washington University estimated in 2010[9] that the total annual cost to a woman of being obese was $8,365* And that's the *annual* cost. Much of this is from higher medical bills for all the obesity-related health issues. Another big chunk is from missing work due to those same health issues—and eventually from premature death.

If you're reading this book, you probably don't need us to convince you of any of this. According to Gallup surveys, the majority of Americans want to lose weight—and this has been true for decades.[10] A vast industry has developed to help us lose these unhealthy extra pounds, and virtually every conceivable diet has been proposed and promoted as a cure. Almost all of these revolve around eliminating something from our diet—and usually something we like. The gluten-free avoid breads, pastas, and most other grains. The paleo attempt to eat only what our distant ancestors may have consumed. Others eschew carbs, fats, sugar, or meat.

Each of these diets has its enthusiasts, and undoubtedly each works for some people. But most of us find the complex rules hard to follow, at least for any prolonged period. The demands of jobs and family make these diets doubly difficult. We're so stressed most days, we don't have time to count calories or study the fine print of ingredients lists. Our lives are complicated enough. We don't need a complicated diet.

And worse, traditional diets can often feel like a punishment. Many of the things we're told to avoid are the ones we

---

* The cost to men was less—which is annoying, although maybe not surprising. But looked at another way, this means the financial benefits of losing weight are higher for women than for men.

most enjoy eating. This may actually be part of what makes those diets work for a while, tricking ourselves into eating less by making it so much less fun. The foods we love become relegated to guilty pleasures. Or they become rewards for good behavior, and leave us constantly judging ourselves and asking what we deserve to eat. Meals become exercises in deprivation rather than nourishment.

This diet takes a different approach. What the Buddha called avoiding untimely eating and those scientists called time-restricted feeding, we call *Buddha's Diet*. Rather than regimenting exactly what you eat, we focus on *when* you eat it. We don't take it to the extreme of fasting after noon like Buddha's monks, but we require you limit your eating to nine hours each day—more like those lucky mice.

The rest of this book will help you understand and practice Buddha's Diet in your own life. Part 1, "Insights," gives you the basic background to understand what Buddha's Diet is all about. In Buddhism, insight (*vipasyana* in Sanskrit) usually means understanding reality, and is the first step on the path to liberation. That's true for dieting, too—the first step is to understand why we get overweight in the first place. We'll say a bit more about those California mice and the revolutionary research behind our timely approach to eating. We'll explain why limiting your meals to certain hours will help you lose weight and how this style of eating actually changes and heals your metabolism.

Part 2, "Practices," explains how to go about the diet itself.

In Buddhism, practices (*sadhana*) are the specific techniques the Buddha taught. They are the nuts and bolts of the Buddha's path, and this part of the book will give you the nuts and bolts of Buddha's Diet. The principles are simple—we've already told you the basics—but they're still a big change for most people. We'll give you a step-by-step plan to make the transition painless and peaceful. We'll also explain what really is known about the science of healthy eating, which is largely the same commonsense notions you've heard all your life—with maybe a few surprises. (If you want to cut to the chase and understand how to start Buddha's Diet *right now*, you can pause here and begin reading chapter 4, "Buddha's Diet.")

Part 3 is called "Hindrances." In the Buddhist tradition, hindrances (*nivarana*) are the mental obstacles that stand in the way of our enlightenment. In dieting, they can be more practical roadblocks. What do I do when I'm hungry? What about eating with my kids? How can I go out on dates without late-night eating and drinking? And what about drinking in general? There are mental blocks to dieting, too. How can I stop eating when I'm stressed? How do I stop treating food as a reward? You probably have lots of questions about the details, and here we'll give you the answers.

Part 4, "Perfections," tells you how Buddha's Diet connects to all the other things the Buddha taught—how to live a healthy, happy, and mindful life. The Buddhist perfections (*paramita*) are the wonderful qualities we each develop as we travel along the path—and we'll show you how to nurture these as you put Buddha's Diet into practice.

Eating should be a joy, not a battle. The Buddha called food one of the four essentials of human existence.[11] Food has an important and necessary place in our lives. Buddha's Diet will help you keep it in that place.

CHAPTER 2

Why Do We Get Fat?

BUDDHA LOVED DATA. MOST RELIGIONS ARE BUILT ON faith, but Buddha emphasized evidence. He wanted us to focus on seeing rather than believing.[1] "Something may be fully accepted out of faith," he preached, "yet it may be empty, hollow, and false."[2]

We've all been told a pretty simple story about why we get fat—we eat too much, or we exercise too little, or maybe both. One way or the other, we consume more calories than we burn, so we gain weight. And we're usually told this as if it's a completely self-evident law of nature.[3]

But what does the evidence say? Medical researchers have been studying this question for decades. They have asked people to eat severely calorie-restricted diets—as little as 800 calories a day, probably *less than half* of what you'll eat today. Yet very few of these poor test subjects have lost weight, and almost none kept it off.[4] Study after study reaches the same conclusion: eating less—even *a lot* less—barely works, and the few pounds you may lose are quickly gained back.

So why *do* we get fat if it isn't overeating? Well, it's a little more complicated.

Your body's metabolism is a very complex machine. It has to be. Think about this basic challenge: your heart, lungs, and brain have to work 24 hours a day, every day of your life, and they need energy—calories—to do that. But even if you're a compulsive snacker—and many of us are—you're not actually eating *constantly*. So where does the energy come from in between? Who's feeding calories to your heart in the middle of the night?

This is why we have fat. There's nothing wrong with fat—you need it for exactly this purpose. Fat is your energy bank. And you'd look terrible without fat, too—like Buddha during that awful emaciated phase. A little fat is a good thing. A lot, not so much.

The number of fat cells you have is determined at birth. Whether you eat Big Macs or salads, you'll have the same number.[5] Molecules of fat go in and out of these cells all day long, supplying energy whenever and wherever it's needed. In a perfect world, our bodies would load up these fat cells during meals, and then slowly drain them the rest of the day and night.[6] They would act like the fuel tank of your car—filled up every so often, then gradually emptied as you drive around.

The problems come when we can't stop filling the tank. When you overfill your car, the tank just overflows and makes a mess. These days, you can't even overfill it if you want to—the pumps just shut off. But your body doesn't have that built-in switch. When you overfill your fat cells, they grow. And grow. You get fat.

Our mitochondria are the tiny power plants of our cells—they take sugar and turn it into actual energy. When there's more sugar in our bloodstream than our cells need, the mitochondria can't keep up. Instead, the fat cells start filling up. This is all controlled by insulin, the hormone that signals for this whole process to get going. Insulin tells your cells to fill up those fat cells instead of draining them.*

Insulin is released whenever you eat sugar, or something (like simple carbohydrates) that can be easily digested into sugar. (It's even released when you *think* about eating sugar, just to get the body ready.) So as long as you're eating sugar, you'll be pumping out lots of insulin. And as long as you're pumping out lots of insulin, you'll be loading up your fat cells. Your body just doesn't have a choice—you won't burn fat as long as there's insulin ordering your cells to store it up.

If we only eat sugar now and then, we're usually fine. The problem is, if we eat too much, too often, we start to accumulate a lot of excess fat. And ironically, all this fat makes our bodies resistant to insulin. This increases the sugar in our blood, and triggers us to pump out even more insulin, which signals our cells to store even more fat, which then makes us

---

* Insulin does a lot of other things, too, but its role in regulating blood sugar is what matters most to us here.

even fatter and even more insulin-resistant.[7] The downward spiral continues unless we take some sort of drastic action.

There's no way to stop eating sugar—almost all food has some. But in most natural food, that sugar is bound up with things like protein, fiber, and water.[8] Unfortunately, our modern diet is filled with processed foods in which much of that buffer is stripped out, and lots of extra sugar is added in. This causes serious problems. In a groundbreaking study of obese children conducted at the University of California, San Francisco, a team of scientists led by Dr. Robert Lustig found that reducing the added sugar in kids' diets by about two-thirds *for just 10 days* significantly improved their insulin sensitivity and other measures of metabolic health.[9] This was without changing their total calorie intake, and with "intensive efforts" to *prevent* weight loss.

What does any of this tell us about Buddha's Diet? The bottom line is this: if we're getting fat because all that sugar is overworking our metabolism and leaving our poor mitochondria unable to keep up, then somehow we need to give our cells a break.

One approach, of course, would be to eat a lot less sugar and simple carbohydrates. This was the approach of that 10-day UCSF study. Several popular sugar-free or no-carb diets recommend just that, and claim good results.[10]

But those mice we met back in the first chapter suggest there's another approach. Maybe what our exhausted metabolism really needs is not a lighter load throughout the day, but the equivalent of a good night's sleep. Instead of asking those mitochondria to work a little less hard 24/7, we could give them some real time off. That's what Buddha's Diet does. This seems to be nature's approach, too. If you look out in the wild, you'll find very few examples of animals getting fat—at least not without good reason.[11] Bears will put on weight before they go into hibernation, but then they'll lose it again over the winter. Squirrels are much the same.[12] When animals gain weight, it usually isn't just because there's extra food around—it's because they want to, or need to. Their bodies are in control of their weight—not the other way around.

And when you think about it, most of these animals also eat on a fairly strict schedule. Animals live on a circadian clock. If they're nocturnal—like raccoons—they'll eat only at night. If they're diurnal—like those squirrels—they'll eat during the day. But you don't see squirrels grabbing a midnight snack, even when they live in a peaceful suburb where there's plenty of food and hardly any predators. And you don't see raccoons getting takeout from your trash cans during the day, even when it would be perfectly safe to do so. They seem programmed to eat at a certain time—and even when there's food galore, they don't seem to get obese the way we do.

Now there are exceptions to this. As we saw with those famous mice, if we let them eat high-sugar foods any time they want, they quickly lose control of their weight. The addictive power of sugar seems so strong that it can over-whelm their natural rhythms. They needed those scientists to force them to stop eating for a while each day in order to keep their weight under control.

You don't have anyone monitoring your diet full-time, so you have to do it yourself. And while you might be able to mimic those mice and eat junk for 10 hours a day and still lose weight, it's honestly a lot harder to do it that way. Sugar and carbs are so addictive that you'll likely find yourself craving more, and that will leave you tempted to cheat. It's like an alcoholic trying to stay sober at a bar—certainly possible, but a lot harder than it needs to be.

You don't have to banish these tasty foods altogether, but Buddha's Diet is easier if you cut down on them, and follow some basic guidelines we'll explain soon. But first, let's delve a bit deeper into the research on those dieting mice.

CHAPTER 3

Eating Like a Mouse

IT'S VERY HARD TO DO GOOD SCIENCE ON DIET AND WEIGHT loss. If you ask people about their diet, they don't tell the whole truth. One study of men and women who had struggled with dieting found that they underestimated their calorie consumption almost 50%![1] And if you tell people to stick to a certain way of eating for any prolonged period, they usually don't follow the instructions exactly. This makes it very hard for scientists to collect solid data. For example, scientists thought for years that eating many small meals instead of three large ones helped people lose weight. But when they accounted for all the misreporting by their subjects, they found the exact opposite.[2]

Worst of all, the gold standard of science—the randomized double-blind study—is almost impossible in dietary research. When scientists want to test out a new drug, they take a group of carefully selected volunteers and give half of them the real drug and half of them a placebo—and they don't tell anyone who's who, including most of the researchers working on the study. But if you try to do that with diets, you run into all sorts of problems. First, it's much harder to get a group of volunteers to change the way they eat for weeks or months than it is to get them to take a few pills every day. Unless the volunteers are monitored 24/7, there's a pretty good chance they'll eventually cheat—and then probably not admit it.

Second, *the volunteers will know they're on a diet*. You can't really ask people to eat less, or stop eating carbs, or start eating paleo, or really change much of anything about their diet without them knowing it. You might think this wouldn't matter, but lots of research over the years shows that it does. Maybe the volunteers have friends who tried gluten-free and didn't lose weight, so they are subtly less motivated to follow the rules. Or the opposite—maybe they believe in the diet so much that they unconsciously make other changes in their lives that help it succeed. These things happen all the time in scientific studies, and they make the results very hard to interpret accurately.

So how do scientists get around all these obstacles? How do they get people to stick to their experimental diets without knowing that they're doing it? For the most part, they don't. They study mice and rats instead.

These little rodents are much more cooperative. And they don't have nosy neighbors who've already sworn off paleo or cleanses or whatever else you're trying to study. Of course, some diets are hard to study in mice or other animals because they won't necessarily eat all the same foods we do. But one great advantage of Buddha's Diet and other time-based approaches is that they are very easy to study this way. If you want to see what happens when mice only eat for 9 hours a day, you just take away the food at other times.

Is it wrong to manipulate our animal friends this way? It's hard to know quite what Buddha would think. He did not impose any blanket prohibition on using animals for practical purposes, at least for laypeople. There is even a popular story of Buddha's rebirth as a rabbit who offers his own body as food for a local priest.[3] He didn't consider animals to be on the same plane as humans—in fact, rebirth in the animal realm was seen as the unhappy consequence of some difficult past karma and was understood to involve more suffering than a human would expect. At the same time, he preached *avihimsa*, or noncruelty, to all sentient beings, including animals. "Not by harming life does one become noble," he said, "one is termed noble for being gentle to all living things."[4] It seems safe to say that Buddha would insist that research animals were treated as humanely as possible, and used only to alleviate the causes of significant human suffering. Sadly, our obesity epidemic would seem to qualify in this regard.

One of the first things scientists learned in these experiments was that time-restricted feeding seems to prevent mice from getting obese in the first place. We already discussed some of Dr. Satchidananda Panda's studies at the Salk Institute in "Of Mice and Monks." Ordinary mice who are given unlimited access to high-fat foods get fat. When instead the food is offered only for nine hours a day, consistent with their natural feeding cycle, the mice seem to eat the same number of calories, but they don't gain weight.[5] They also don't run into all the metabolic problems that plague the fat mice.

It's a little harder to study actual weight *loss* in mice, because mice aren't naturally fat to begin with. You have to help them gain weight. To do this, the Salk Institute researchers started the mice on the all-you-can-eat high-fat diet for 13 weeks, then switched them to the time-restricted diet for 12 weeks.[6] Sure enough, the mice gained considerable weight during the first phase, but then lost 5% on average when they limited their eating hours again. That's like a 160-pound person losing eight pounds—equivalent to a pound dropped for every week and a half of dieting. Mice who were kept on the unrestricted diet for 26 weeks and then switched to a time-restricted diet lost even more—12% over 12 weeks—presumably because they got more obese at the start. That's like going from 160 pounds down to 141 in under three months.

A few studies of time-restricted diets have been done using actual people. Since the rules are so much simpler than they are for many other diets, it's a bit easier to get reliable volunteers, although you still can't make the tests "blind"—everyone knows when they're eating and when they aren't. Happily, though, the studies that have been done have come out well for this time-restricted approach. For example, on one study of 29 young men, eliminating all nighttime eating for just two weeks caused them to lose about a pound on average.[7] Again, that's about half a pound per week—and they allowed a full 13 hours of eating, considerably more than we recommend on Buddha's Diet. In another study, a group of normal-weight, middle-aged adults were asked to restrict their eating to a 4-hour (!) period for 8 weeks.[8] They lost an average of 3 pounds on this fairly extreme diet, or a bit under a half pound per week—perhaps less than you'd expect, but this may be because none of them was overweight to start with.

More recently, Dr. Panda has also moved from mice to men—and women. He and his colleagues recruited a small group of overweight adults to use a smartphone app to track their eating throughout the day by taking photos of everything they ate. They then asked these volunteers to limit their eating to 10–12 hours—all of whom previously had been eating for at least 14 hours a day. They asked them to keep this up for 16 weeks, without making any other suggestions about diet or nutrition changes, and weighed everyone before and after. Sure enough, almost everyone lost weight, with an average loss of over 7 pounds (or about half a pound per week again). Not only that, but everyone in the study expressed an interest in staying on the diet, and they maintained their weight loss after a full year.[9]

Taken together, the scientific evidence is pretty clear: limiting your eating to certain hours will help you lose weight.

In the next chapter, we'll tell you how to make this way of eating work for you.

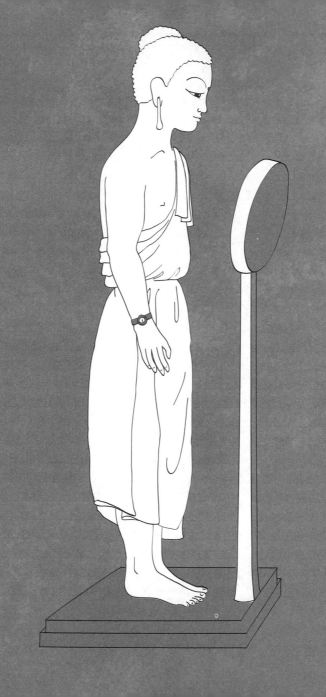

PART 2

PRACTICES

CHAPTER 4

Buddha's Diet

DR. PANDA'S SMARTPHONE STUDY DID MORE THAN PROVE that Buddha's Diet works—it also shed light on how Americans actually eat. If you ask people about their diet, they'll probably tell you they eat three meals a day, with maybe occasional snacks scattered in between. But when Dr. Panda looked at all the photos people took of their food, he found something else entirely: people pretty much eat all day long.[1]

Many of the subjects in the trial ate more than a dozen times a day. The median time from first meal to last was almost 15 hours—meaning that half the people ate for even longer than that every day! Only about 10% initially ate for 12 hours or less.

There's nothing particularly natural about this modern habit of eating all the time. If you've ever been camping, you've probably had the experience of trying to cook in the dark. It's no fun at all—and cleaning up after is even worse. Now imagine trying to do the same thing without flashlights or electric lanterns, with just the flicker of the fire and maybe the faint glow of an oil lamp. It suddenly becomes a whole lot of work to make yourself a late-evening dinner, and almost impossible to whip up a midnight snack.

Before industrial times, people didn't do all that much after dark because, well, it was too dark. In northern India, where the Buddha lived, there was often less than eleven hours of daylight each day—and as little as five hours of bright sun. People had to squeeze in not just eating, but cooking, cleaning, dressing, washing, planting, harvesting, and just about everything else during those hours. And these folks had it easy compared to the countless generations who lived before human agriculture—those poor souls had to hunt and kill their food during those same few hours, too. Many of them probably ate the way lions and tigers and our other carnivore cousins do in the wild—not even every day, let alone all day long.[2]

So when Buddha insisted that monks not eat after noon, he was certainly suggesting a change, but not quite as radical a change as it might seem today. The idea that we should eat sporadically across all our waking hours is not much older than the lightbulb, and is certainly not how humans originally evolved to eat. In evolutionary terms, it might as well have happened yesterday—and in countries like Burma, Thailand, and Sri Lanka, hundreds of thousands of Buddhist monks still follow the Buddha's strict eating schedule every day.

With Buddha's Diet, we return to something more like that original style of eating, and we give our metabolisms the same nice, long break each night that our ancestors did. It may feel unnatural at first, but everyone on earth used to eat this way—and almost all of the animal kingdom still does.

We all know that bad habits can be hard to break, and for many people bad eating habits are harder than most. So we recommend a gradual approach. You don't have to change your whole eating routine overnight—just follow these few steps, and in a short time, you'll be on Buddha's Diet.

STEP 0: ROUND-THE-CLOCK EATING

Step 0 is where you are now, your baseline, and probably the reason you're reading this book in the first place. Our goal is to have you out of Step 0 very quickly. Today, actually. As we've discussed, round-the-clock eating, in the mindless style many of us consider normal, is not normal at all. Unfortunately in many parts of the world—and the United States in particular—cheap, easily accessible, and poor quality food is ready and waiting for us 24/7. This diagram illustrates the unfortunate, modern norm for eating in this country, with meals and snacks consumed throughout the day:

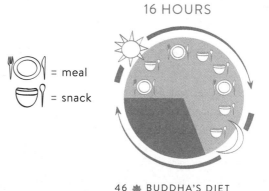

16 HOURS

= meal

= snack

In looking at this diagram you may be thinking: That's ridiculous, I don't eat for 16 hours! Really? Think about it. Remember, everything counts. Just because you aren't having a meal, doesn't mean you aren't eating. Do you have a snack while watching TV before bed? Do you finish your glass of wine an hour before you turn in for the night? All that counts. Now that you notice your current eating clock is way too generous, it's time to move to start dialing it back.

STEP 1: THE 12-HOUR WINDOW

The first true step of Buddha's Diet is to confine your eating to 12 hours a day. Don't worry about changing what you eat or how much you eat—just do it all within 12 hours. The most natural schedule for most people is something like 7 a.m. to 7 p.m. or 8 a.m. to 8 p.m., but choose a window that works for you. If you work an early shift, maybe you need to have breakfast at 6 a.m. If you're a late-riser (or a college student), maybe you want to start your eating day at 10:00 a.m. or 10:30 a.m.—but try not to let it get too late. There is some evidence that eating late at night can be problematic, especially when you're trying to lose weight.[3] We don't know exactly why this is, but it may be that the body has a harder time dealing with all those calories when your metabolism is operating out of sync with your circadian rhythm. (This is especially tricky if you have to work a night shift. Recent studies suggest nighttime work and daytime sleep makes weight loss more challenging,[4] in part because the body seems to burn calories differently when you sleep during the day.)

Whatever window you choose, make sure you finish dinner (and eating—so dessert, snacks, *everything*) within 12 hours from the start of breakfast, as this diagram shows:

12 HOURS

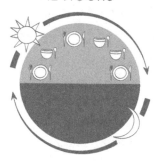

Keep in mind that while we include snacks in the 12-hour window diagram, you don't *have* to snack. More than likely though, you are snacking during these hours—maybe even a lot. But how many meals and snacks you eat is up to you at this point. We are focused on the *when*, not the *how much* or the *what*. A lot of people don't need to adjust any meal times to make this work, but you do have to stop nighttime nibbling.

One thing you may notice at this step is just how much you used to eat *after* dinner. In the smartphone study, participants ate over a *third* of their calories after 6 p.m.—and almost all of those were probably unnecessary. As the scientists put it in precise technical terms, "food consumed after 6:36 p.m.

exceeded the maintenance calories requirement."[5] Whether it's popcorn while you stream a movie or a cocktail on the couch, you may be surprised by how much you used to consume in the evening. All of this has to stop. (And yes, drinking counts. We have a whole chapter on this coming up.)

In many ways, this first step is both the easiest and the hardest. It's easy because many of us don't even need to reschedule any of our real meals—or we need to shift them only very little—to squeeze them into 12 hours. But it's hard because we have to pay attention to when we're eating, and we have to train ourselves to stop, completely, when our time is up. You'll probably find that a lot of what you were eating after dinner was of the empty calories variety, or just plain old junk food. Almost no one whips up a kale salad or a roast when they're craving a snack at 11 p.m.—we grab ice cream or chips or something else easy, processed, and often unhealthy. A side benefit of minimizing your eating hours in the evening is you simply won't reach for so much of that stuff anymore. There may be a few nights at first when you can't imagine you'll make it until morning without a snack. But you will.

How long should you be on this step? We recommend staying on each step for two weeks. For some, two weeks is too aggressive. This may be especially true if you have family or job responsibilities that need to be adjusted to make this work. *But only move to the next step when you've stayed on this schedule for two weeks straight with no more than one "cheat day" per week.* If that takes you four weeks, that's okay, too.

Buddha spent years as a wandering ascetic before discovering his middle way. Success is more important than speed. Soon this will all become second nature. Remember that you are forming new patterns and with them a new eating clock.

You may start losing weight as soon as you get to Step 1—in fact, the harder this step is for you, the more likely it will lead to immediate weight loss. Although weight loss usually starts slowly, a realistic goal is to lose between half a pound and a pound per week on Buddha's Diet, just as we saw in those studies in the previous chapter. This may not sound like much, but keep in mind that you're in this for the long haul. And you're creating a brand-new eating mind-set that will serve you for a lifetime. Even half a pound per week could add up to twenty pounds this year. (And we have a whole chapter on weighing yourself next.)

STEP 2: THE 11-HOUR WINDOW

The next step is to start shrinking your eating window. We'll start by reducing it by an hour—to 11 instead of 12. Where you want to take that hour from is up to you. For some people, the easiest way to do this is to push breakfast an hour later. If you were eating 7 a.m. to 7 p.m., try 8 a.m. to 7p.m. instead. If you exercise in the mornings, postpone breakfast until after that. If you go straight to work, maybe you can bring breakfast with you and make it a midmorning break once you get settled. At first you'll probably be hungry in the mornings, but this is more from habit than biological need. The other option is to take that hour from the evening, bumping up dinner an hour earlier. In general, we will be moving in that direction anyway, toward less food in the evenings, so trying it out now will give you a preview of the next step in the diet. It may feel strange to shave this time off your eating schedule at first. But you're not going to starve. Unless you are already skeletally thin, you have more than enough reserves to get you through that extra hour.

Again, your goal is to stay on this step for two weeks before moving on to the next. Nobody is perfect, and we understand that everyone will slip up now and then. There's even some reason to believe a little bit of "cheating" on a diet can be healthy. (We have a chapter on that coming up.) But if you're having more than one cheat day a week, you haven't mastered the step. Too many cheat days equals erratic eating. And erratic eating means you've landed yourself back in Step 0.

Once you've successfully mastered Step 2, your meal schedule looks like this (assuming you've taken that hour from the evening):

11 HOURS

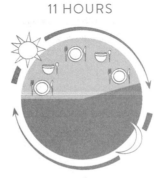

Note that a few people have serious medical issues that require them to spread their eating over more than 11 hours. Some people get migraines if they don't eat as soon as they wake up. Others may have to titrate their blood sugar carefully and eat lots of small meals to keep it in range. If you have a medical need to eat at certain times, you should certainly talk to your doctor before making any changes. Even the Buddha made exceptions for monks who were ill.

STEP 3: THE 10-HOUR WINDOW

Now you're ready to take things a bit further and reduce your eating down to 10 hours. To do this, you probably need to shift both your breakfast and your dinner—possibly all three meals. We don't recommend shortening your eating window by skipping breakfast altogether and eating, say, between noon and 10 p.m. Again, there just seems to be something especially challenging for our bodies about late-night eating—outside our natural circadian rhythm—and it is often harder to make good food choices then, too.* So your best bet is stopping earlier in the day and not starting later.

You will probably find that with your meals spaced more closely together, you don't need to snack like you used to. Squeezing three meals into 10 hours means your meals are

* There are some conflicting studies on late-night eating, probably in part because people who eat late also have different sleep patterns, which also affects their weight. But the tendency to binge-eat at night is well established, and there are no studies suggesting it's a good idea.

rarely more than three hours apart. This makes it much less likely that you'll get hungry in between—and if you do, the next meal is coming up so soon that you can just wait.

The 10-hour window can be challenging, especially if you've been used to eating a lot outside of these hours. Even if the other steps have been relatively easy, this may be the one that takes more than two weeks to get right. Don't worry too much about that—you will master the step, just as you've mastered the others. It may simply take a bit longer.

You may find there are plenty of times when the 10-hour window is particularly difficult—maybe you are putting in long hours at work or you find yourself needing to have a later dinner because a child has soccer practice in the evening or you're going out. How do you pull off the 10-hour window then? It's actually not as challenging as you might think, and we address many of these hurdles specifically in later chapters. The truth is, life will never be perfectly aligned to follow any diet, ever. You will have slipups now and then— we all do. A little bit of cheating isn't the end of the world. But you can still get to your weight loss goals a lot faster, more enjoyably, and more consistently if you try your best to stick to these eating windows as many days as you can. And like the other steps, you need to be on the schedule for at least two weeks with no more than one cheat day each week to continue.

One thing you can do as you are planning your hours is to consider what your life is like at this very moment. For example, it's probably not a great idea to start this diet over the holidays, when you'll be expected to join lots of big, late dinners or parties, and not ideal to start when adjusting to a new work routine, either. While Buddha's Diet isn't nearly as restrictive as some (a carb-free Thanksgiving can be pretty depressing) it's still one more thing to take on during a busy and stressful time when eating schedules are often disrupted.

But once you start the 10-hour window, you'll find that soon enough you'll adjust, and after a while, you won't think much about the diet at all because it will have become second nature.

This leaves us with an eating schedule that looks like this:

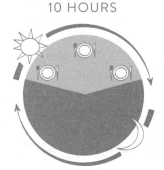

STEP 4: THE 9-HOUR WINDOW

You will have noticed weight loss in Step 3, especially if you were eating well outside the 10-hour window before. If you are already seeing good results, you may want to stay on that schedule for a few extra weeks and see if that weight loss continues at the rate you hope. However, the goal of this diet and the way to reap the most benefits is by reducing to nine hours, giving you a schedule that looks like this:

9 HOURS

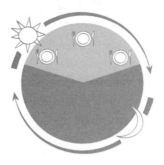

One thing you'll likely find with a 9-hour eating window is that you don't need to eat as much at dinner. This seems counterintuitive—after all, this dinner has to last you 15 hours until breakfast! But you'll be asleep much of that time, and your body will naturally slow down. Because dinner will now inevitably be closer to lunch, you just won't be as hungry. (Of course, what you eat at these meals will also affect how hungry you are—and a chapter on "What to Eat" is coming up.)

Whatever you do, resist the temptation to load up on extra food because you're worried about being hungry later. You're not a bear going into hibernation—you have a good breakfast coming in the morning. Eat only what you feel you need *right now*, and you may find that the hunger you were worried about never comes.

The other nice thing about the 9-hour window is that there's a little more room for error. Maybe despite your best intentions, you just can't get dinner made and eaten in time. Or you have an early meeting and just have to eat breakfast before you get to work. Or maybe you're at home with sick kids all day and you're just trying to survive. If you miss your deadline by a bit on this schedule, you'll still be well within the 10-hour window—likely a huge improvement on your old eating habits.

Once you're on the nine-hour window, you're on Buddha's Diet. Congratulations, you've done it. You are what Buddha might call a *sottapana*, a "stream-enterer." It is now only a matter of time before you reach your weight loss goal.

Not only that, but you will have also changed your eating habits. Forever. That mindless grazing you used to do at night? Gone. The thoughtless snacking throughout the day to combat boredom and stress? Finished. The all-hours buffet of bad choices? Over. Your mind has undergone a change as much as your body has. You'll see this in the form of greater discipline, more selective choices, and increased mindfulness about eating. When the hours and the things you eat take on increased importance, it quickly becomes easier to move away forever from the free-for-all foraging of your old life.

There are people out there who advocate even smaller eating windows than 9 hours. One recent book suggests six,[6] while other studies have even limited participants to a single meal.[7] And, of course, there are all those actual monks, eating only between dawn and noon. But in the spirit of the middle way, we feel that the 9-hour window of Buddha's Diet represents the right balance. It *is* a change, and leads to some obstacles that the next part of the book will address. But at the same time, it's entirely doable. Pushing your breakfast a little later and eating an earlier dinner isn't *that* hard. Before the modern era, just about everyone did it. You can, too.

CHAPTER 5

What Did Buddha Weigh?

HOW MUCH DID BUDDHA WEIGH? WE HAVE NO IDEA. HE didn't know, either. Although simple balance scales have been around just about forever, they were primarily for commercial trade. As someone who started life as a prince and ended it as a monk, Buddha may not have personally bought or sold anything his whole life.

It's not clear that anyone paid much attention to their own precise weight until modern times. No one *could* care much about their weight until "penny scales" started appearing in drugstores and groceries in the late 1800s.[1] Smaller bathroom scales emerged a few decades later.[2] Pretty soon, everyone wanted to know their own weight.

We don't want you to become obsessed with the number you see on the scale. Your weight is not your worth. But if you don't already weigh yourself regularly, you should start doing this now. In fact, you should weigh yourself every day. *Every day.*

Why every day? Well, your goal is to eliminate as many variables as you can. Your weight fluctuates day to day and hour to hour, whether you're trying to lose weight or not. A 16-ounce coffee weighs almost exactly a pound. If you weigh yourself one morning before your coffee and one morning after, guess what? Your weight will be different. Your breakfast, your clothes, your phone—they all weigh something. And if you're trying to measure a change of half a pound over a week, that's just a little more than an ounce per day—a lot less than the iPhone you might have forgotten to put down. If you always sleep in the same pajamas, you can leave those on if you'd like. But two different T-shirts can have different weights by as much as several ounces, even if they are supposedly the same size. So weigh yourself at the same time every day, wear the same clothes (or none at all), and use the same scale. It's as simple as that.

When is the best time to weigh yourself? Right after you get up is fine, and easy to remember. If you're someone who starts off in the bathroom anyway, you can do it right then. Just before your shower is good, too, since you're already undressed—as long as you generally shower at the same time each day, and preferably before eating breakfast. But if your mornings are too rushed and unpredictable as it is, just weighing yourself first thing will work, too.

What's the point of all this weighing? It's simple: There is lots of evidence that weighing yourself regularly helps you lose weight. In a recent survey of 17 scientific studies of weight monitoring and weight management, self-weighing proved helpful in all of them.[3] In one two-year study, adults who weighed themselves daily lost weight, while those who weighed themselves only monthly added pounds.[4] Obviously getting on and off the scale is not in itself burning many calories, but literally watching your weight helps you become aware of how your diet and life impact your body.

This is essential. A big part of Buddha's Diet is learning how your daily rhythm of eating is impacting your weight. Without measuring your weight, you're missing vital data to help you make these connections. Some used to worry that all this time on the scale might make people discouraged or depressed, but more recent research hasn't shown evidence of this.[5] As one study put it, these daily weighings let you "catch and reverse small weight gains" along the way, so you stay on track.[6]

For some this may seem obsessive. Every day? Are we really defined by a number? Of course not. Eventually when you have attained your goal and you are adhering to your eating clock without any trouble, you can cut back on the weighing considerably. (We have a chapter on that weight maintenance phase later in the book.) You may put on a few pounds during the holidays (it's very hard to not eat after a certain hour when all around you are celebrations and eating), but with Buddha's Diet you can easily get back on track—and that will naturally happen once the festivities conclude. Your daily ups and downs won't matter as much.

Our weight can give us crucial clues. Doctors know this, of course. Often the first thing you do in a doctor's office is step on the scale. It may seem like a simple thing, but this number can give your doctor a sense of a trend. Have you gained weight at the last three appointments? Maybe there's more than a consumption problem—maybe there's a medical issue. Or conversely, maybe you keep losing weight—enough that your doctor wonders if maybe there's something more serious going on, either physical or emotional.

In the same way your doctor may want to track your blood pressure, your cholesterol, and other vital markers, weight can be valuable data. The number, whatever it is, doesn't make you a good or a bad person, a weak or a strong person. It's just a number that can give insight—insight you can use to refine and perfect Buddha's Diet.

Weighing yourself daily is a way of taking control over your diet and health. Just as Buddha wanted proof he could see with his own eyes, this daily ritual will help you gather data about what is and isn't working. Did those two cheat days hurt, or barely make a difference? Did cutting a half hour from your eating window help you drop a bit from one day to the next? You won't know if you aren't getting on the scale.

As with so much of Buddha's Diet, the trick is to pay attention to your weight, *but not too much attention*. Even if you are very consistent about your weighing rituals, there are still going to be inevitable ups and downs that don't necessarily mean anything. Our weight isn't constant. It's most important to focus on patterns that stretch across several days, or even weeks. The easiest way to do this is with a networked scale that talks to your phone or tablet. It may seem like a gimmick, but it will draw you a nice chart that shows your weight over time and let you see the long-term direction. If you don't want to spend that much, there are also lots of apps that will show you those same averages and charts after you enter your daily weight manually. If you're brave, these apps will even let you share your data with a friend or two, to help motivate each other to stick to your goals. However you manage it, don't focus *too* much on any one day's weight. Focus on trends over multiple days and weeks, and you'll soon find yourself approaching your goal.

Although most of us would much prefer to weigh ourselves in private these days, those old-fashioned public scales still exist here and there. Several antiques still stand in the great Luxembourg Garden in Paris. The originals were inscribed with a simple motto, which translates roughly to this: "He who often weighs himself, knows himself well. He who knows himself well, lives well."[7]

You can certainly live well without knowing your weight. But tracking your weight really does help you know yourself better. It will teach you how your body responds to food, and put you in control of that relationship.

CHAPTER 6

What to Eat

IF YOU LOOK AROUND THE WORLD, YOU'LL SEE INCREDIBLE variety in what people eat. There are diets based almost exclusively on meat, and diets that are strictly vegetarian. There are cultures that consume mostly protein or fat or grain. There are cuisines based on rice, on wheat, on corn, or on potatoes. And there is huge variation in how much people eat. One survey of world diets found ordinary people consuming anywhere from 800 to 12,300 calories per day![1]

There may be some biological differences between these populations—some groups like the Tibetans may have been genetically isolated for so long that their metabolisms have evolved a bit differently from everyone else's. But the bottom line is that human beings seem able to survive and thrive on a huge range of foods.

There are no hard and fast rules about what to eat on Buddha's Diet. It's most important to eat food you like and find filling. The biggest problem with restrictive diets is not necessarily that they don't work, but that hardly anyone can stick to them. A diet that makes you miserable is not one that is going to last.

And as we've explained before, Buddha himself didn't provide much guidance on what to eat. Like all monks, he basically ate whatever local people offered him. There are a few provisions about not *asking* for rich or fancy foods—but monks were permitted to eat them if they were freely given. Monks weren't encouraged to take more food than they needed or to shuffle food around in their bowls to make it look like they didn't have enough. About the only food label you can really put on Buddha is "locavore," since all his food came from his daily alms rounds, conducted entirely on foot.

It's not that India was devoid of picky eaters. Just like today, devout Brahmins in Buddha's time followed complex rules around food and drink. They were fastidious vegetarians, who also avoided eggs, onions, and garlic. They even refrained from eating mushrooms, believing they were "unclean" because they grow on dung (which does sound pretty gross when you think about it). There were other even stricter diets around—including some that prohibited eating anything stale or overripe or anything with the wrong flavors or texture. And there were stringent rules about which castes could accept which foods from other castes, something Buddha didn't like at all. (He dropped all caste distinctions among his followers.)

Buddha may have been reacting against these persnickety diets when he decreed that monks and nuns should just eat whatever they received. He would likely be disheartened by the multitude of restrictive diets we have today—no carbs, gluten-free, paleo, and all that. He didn't want his followers getting too wrapped up in what exactly they ate. He wanted us to treat food as the vital sustenance it is, and leave it at that.

Our advice then is less about what foods are *good* or *bad* and more about what foods are *useful*. We already reviewed the role of sugar in obesity in "Why Do We Get Fat?" so it won't come as any surprise that we recommend you limit it. The biggest problem with sugar on Buddha's Diet is that it makes you hungry. There's a reason it's so hard to eat just one cookie, or just a smidgen of ice cream. All that sugar triggers a rush of insulin, and then all that insulin makes you want more sugar. It's not so much that sugar is unhealthy as that it's *unhelpful*.

Of course, for many of us, cutting down on sugar is much easier said than done. Scientists have found that our general preference for sweetness is "both innate and universal," but at the same time, our preferences for sweetness in specific foods can change over time.[2] Sensory researchers find that each of us has a *bliss point*, "the precise amount of sweetness—no more, no less—that makes food and drink most enjoyable."[3] But this point shifts over time. For example, when researchers prepare solutions with various concentrations of sugar dissolved in water, they find that children and adolescents prefer sweeter concoctions than adults.[4]

As we've discussed earlier, the bad news about sugar is that the more you eat, the more you want. Our bodies habituate to sweet taste the same way they do to drugs, so that it quickly takes even more sweetness to elicit the same response.[5] Most of us have become addicted to all the added sugar in our diets.

The good news is that you can turn this cycle around: over time the less sugar you eat, the less you want, too. Your bliss point will shift down, and you'll find you need much less sugar to enjoy your foods and drinks as much as before. Try putting half as much sugar in your coffee or tea for a couple weeks, and your old way of drinking it will soon taste too sweet.

Similarly, if you look at centuries past, many spices we take for granted now were either unknown to most of the world or were incredible luxuries. Black pepper is native to South and Southeast Asia and had to be brought by ship across the Indian Ocean to reach Europe. It was not cheap. Even salt was costly if you didn't live close enough to seawater to dry your own. Whole empires in Europe were funded by the salt trade. We evolved in an age when all these tastes were very scarce and it was fine to eat as much as you could when you found them. So it's no big surprise that our bodies don't always respond in a healthy way to the modern reality of abundance.

We all have foods we can't stop eating, even when we aren't hungry. Pay attention to how you respond to different foods.

Processed foods are often the toughest—they are designed to be addictive. A study at the University of Michigan asked nearly 400 volunteers which foods were associated with classic addiction behaviors—things like not being able to stop, using despite knowing the negative consequences, and triggering withdrawal symptoms.[6] The top seven on this addictive scale were pizza, chocolate, chips, cookies, ice cream, french fries, and cheeseburgers—all processed foods. (If that list doesn't make you hungry, you may not need this book.) The bottom scorers were carrots and cucumbers. As the researchers summarize, "an unprocessed food, such as an apple, is less likely to trigger an addictive-like response than a highly processed food, such as a cookie," even though both contain sugar. The cookie takes the sugar, combines it with fat, and delivers it into our bloodstream much more quickly than a fruit would—effectively turning a natural ingredient into a drug.

This means for most of us, if our last meal of the day is a bag of potato chips, we're asking for trouble. First, we'll probably eat more than we mean to—likely the whole bag, and maybe even the next bag if it's right there. And second, even if we make ourselves stop, we'll get hungry again quickly, because our body will digest all that starch in a hurry and be left wanting more. Waiting until breakfast to eat again is going to be a struggle.

As you embark on Buddha's Diet, you'll learn your body's own tricks and quirks. For most people, protein does a better job of filling us up than simple carbohydrates.[7] It also takes more energy to digest proteins. Fat has similar properties. In one study, when subjects added some fat to their food (without changing the total calories), they naturally delayed their next meal by more than half an hour.[8] The fat just kept them full longer. Similarly, food with whole grains and fiber seems to fill us up better than foods made from refined flours and starches. In another study, people who ate a high-fiber lunch reported feeling less hungry two and three hours later, and consequently these foods may result in less snacking.[9] On Buddha's Diet, choosing whole grains rather than refined carbohydrates will keep you full longer and make you less inclined to cheat.

These guidelines for meals apply to snacks, too—high-protein snacks are the best way to fight hunger, and high-carb snacks are the worst.[10] Another thing to keep in mind: don't snack when you're not hungry. Maybe that seems obvious, but research has shown that eating a snack when you're not hungry has no effect at all on what you eat at the next meal.[11] Although some will tell you that eating lots of small meals can help you on a diet, modern controlled studies have found the opposite, that eating less frequently leads to "better body weight control in the long term."[12] Mindlessly grazing during the day is going to be counterproductive. You'll still eat just as much at lunch and dinner, and all those extra calories won't do you any good.

What about drinks? We have another whole chapter on

that coming up, but the shortest advice is that you are generally better off eating your calories than drinking them, in a large part because solid food is just more filling than liquids.[13] And when we drink sugar-sweetened beverages, we don't generally compensate by eating less later, so we end up with more overall calories in the day without any real benefit.

Although true malnutrition is rare in rich countries, there are a few things you'll want to pay attention to. You need calcium for healthy bones and lots of people don't get enough—especially women. Green vegetables like broccoli and collard greens have good amounts of calcium, but the most potent sources are dairy products like milk, cheese, and yogurt, or a commercial supplement. Vitamins are vital to a healthy body and are found in fruits and vegetables, though if you're worried, a daily multivitamin is a nice insurance policy.

What does all this mean about the latest food fad you may have heard about? Should you eat more kale? Or flax seeds? Should you load up on antioxidants? Or omega-3s? The truth is that anyone who answers those questions for you definitively is probably overstating the evidence. The reason even the best scientists don't agree is that the effects of most of these substances is likely subtle and small. Some data suggests antioxidants are good for you.[14] Some suggests they're actually bad.[15] But if they were *very* good or *very* bad, it wouldn't be so hard to prove it one way or the other. In one survey of ingredients chosen at random from an American cookbook, scientists found that fully 80% had been studied for their effect on cancer, with 39% allegedly increasing risk and 33% reducing it. Yet they also found that these claims were largely based on "weak statistical evidence" and noted: "Randomized trials have repeatedly failed to find treatment effects for nutrients in which observational studies had previously proposed strong associations."[16] In science just like in a scavenger hunt, it's much easier to find big things than tiny ones. For a lot of these foods, whatever their effect is, it's likely so small that it's difficult to measure it at all.

If you feel like eating more kale—or if eating more kale seems to make you feel better—by all means, do it. But if you can't stand flax seeds, don't let anyone convince you they are a necessary part of a healthy diet. If you're eating a variety of foods you like, feeling satisfied between meals, and sticking to your schedule every day, you're probably doing just fine. And if you're already on a paleo or gluten-free or low-carb diet and loving it, there's no need to stop. You can keep eating that way if it works for you, as long as you keep to your hours, too. (Bear in mind that if you're a proponent of eating like a caveman, as the paleo diet champions, our distant ancestors weren't able to fix themselves a late-night snack by moonlight, either. So you could see Buddha's Diet as a way to double down on paleo.)

An important benefit of Buddha's Diet is that you're eating your meals at times of the day when you're most likely to make good food choices. It's more common to down a quart of ice cream at midnight than it is at noon—researchers find that almost 70% of all ice cream is consumed after 6 p.m.[17] When we're tired at the end of a long day, we're vulnerable to all sorts of bad feelings and bad decisions. And we might not have time to prepare something healthy, even if we held on to our good intentions. So on Buddha's Diet, we just skip over the temptations altogether, and do our eating at a time when we can do it well.

One last thing to note: there's no need to cut out junk food altogether—and no guarantee that never touching a french fry again will solve your weight woes. A recent study tells us that people in all weight categories consume fast food, soft drinks, and candy.[18] So cut down, but keep your focus on maintaining your eating schedule.

The essential thing is to listen to your body. As you spend more time on Buddha's Diet, you'll naturally gravitate to healthy meals based on protein, fat, and high-fiber grains that don't leave you constantly craving your next food fix. Now that you can no longer eat at random times, your food choices will become less reckless and more thoughtful.

CHAPTER 7

Meat or Potatoes?

AS WE MENTIONED IN "OF MICE AND MONKS," BUDDHA
was not a vegetarian. He and his monks ate whatever local
villagers offered them, which often included meat. Today
most Buddhists are not vegetarian, either—although some
certainly are. But the countries with the oldest Buddhist
traditions, such as Thailand and Sri Lanka, tend to have
the fewest vegetarians. Vegetarianism doesn't seem to have
become part of Buddhism at all until the religion got to
China, centuries after the Buddha's death.[1]

This doesn't mean Buddha didn't care about animals. He
forbid monks from slaughtering their own meat or even asking someone else to do it for them. But he also prohibited
monks from farming, because even working the soil inevitably results in killing countless tiny beings.[2] This was one of
Buddha's great insights—all life involves death.

It wasn't that vegetarianism wasn't discussed. In one story,

Buddha's cousin Devadatta suggested that Buddha prohibit monks from eating meat.[3] To be clear, Devadatta was a bit of a troublemaker,* and it's generally thought that Devadatta was only suggesting a ban on meat so he could appear even holier than the Buddha. "Whoever should eat fish and flesh," he argued, "sin would besmirch him." But Buddha disagreed. "Fish and flesh are pure," he insisted, as long as they were not "seen, heard, or suspected" to have been killed explicitly for the monks. Yet the very fact that Devadatta thought suggesting vegetarianism could make him into a sort of teacher's pet shows that it was seen as something positive and holy, even back then.

These days, the health issues surrounding animal protein are complicated and controversial. For many years, nutritionists recommended severely limiting consumption of saturated fat, which most sources of animal protein have in abundance. But many now feel this was a mistake and that the evidence against saturated fats is lacking.[4] So saturated fat alone may not be a reason to avoid eating meat.

And all the issues that make it hard to study diet and weight loss make it similarly hard to study diet and health. We can't do randomized double-blind studies of vegetarians versus meat eaters, because people know whether they're eating meat or not. (Veggie burgers are getting very good, but they're not yet *that* good.) We can't even really study

---

* Actually, he was a *huge* troublemaker. He tried to kill Buddha— more than once. But Buddha was very forgiving and let him stick around. Remember that when you get annoyed with your own family.

this question in animals, since we can't be sure our bodies would respond in the same way as theirs. Even worse, most of the health effects of a vegetarian diet are likely to arise over the very long term. Maybe you can convince some volunteers to be vegetarians for a few months or even a year, but lots of human health issues take decades to emerge.

Still, we can say with certainty that when we survey the population, vegetarians seem to be healthier than nonvegetarians. They have significantly lower risk of heart disease.[5] The list of health benefits goes on and on from there, including lower blood pressure, fewer gallstones, less diabetes, and reduced risk for dementia.[6] One study in the 1980s found that vegetarian adults followed for 12 years were half as likely to die *for any reason at all* as the general population.[7] And if that's not enough, vegetarians tend to be thinner.[8]

Perhaps most significantly, vegetarians also seem to have fewer cancers.[9] The association between meat eating and cancer is so strong and the evidence is so consistent that the International Agency for Research on Cancer, a division of the World Health Organization, recently concluded that eating processed meat (specifically "meat that has been transformed through salting, curing, fermentation, [or] smoking"—think hot dogs and bacon) definitely causes colorectal cancer, while eating ordinary red meat ("unprocessed mammalian muscle" if you want to get gross about it) "probably" causes colorectal cancer.

Of course, it's possible that vegetarians are just more

health conscious. Perhaps people who go through the trouble of avoiding meat also make other good choices about their lives, or generally care more about the food they eat than the general population. You can be a vegetarian and eat nothing but pizza and ice cream, but it seems most don't go that route (as tempting as it is). But even this last-ditch hope for meat-lovers is getting less and less likely as scientists gradually uncover the actual mechanisms by which eating meat seems to damage our bodies.[10]

Some people used to worry that vegetarians didn't get enough protein, but this no longer seems to be a serious concern. The official position of the American Dietetic Association is that "Plant protein can meet protein requirements when a variety of plant foods is consumed and energy needs are met."[11] In other words, if you're getting enough calories, you're probably getting enough protein, vegetarian or not. Long ago, some people used to insist that you had to eat plants in certain combinations—like beans with corn, or soy with rice—in order to create "complete" proteins, and you still hear people talk about this today. But as far back as 1994, experts were already labeling this a myth,[12] and the concept isn't even mentioned in the most recent FDA nutrition guidelines.[13]

In countries where Buddhists have embraced vegetarianism, however, the potential health benefits generally have nothing to do with it. Rather, these Buddhists feel being a vegetarian is part of honoring Buddha's admonition to cherish all life. They don't want animals to suffer and die unnecessarily. Buddha would no doubt be sympathetic to that. There are many stories of him showing kindness to animals—even a whole series of stories about past lives when he was an animal himself. In one, Buddha is reborn as a deer. When a hunter somehow recognizes his greatness and offers to spare his life, Buddha-the-deer insists he will only accept his mercy if the whole herd is spared. (The hunter agrees.) In another, Buddha is reborn as a fish—and refuses to eat other fish.[14]

Today many vegetarians also cite the environmental cost of raising animals for food. The meat industry produces vastly more carbon emissions than farming the equivalent vegetables.[15] Every type of meat is different, but beef, for example, generates 13 times the emissions per pound compared to plant protein.

Yet despite all this, most people are not vegetarian and aren't likely to make the switch anytime soon. A 2012 Gallup poll found that only about 5% of Americans consider themselves vegetarians, and only 2% consider themselves vegan.[16] Chances are you aren't vegetarian, and aren't going to become one after reading this chapter.

But it doesn't have to be an all-or-nothing thing. The study on heart disease, for example, showed that vegetarians had a 34% lower risk than regular meat eaters—but occasional meat eaters had a 20% lower risk than regular meat eaters, too. So you get most of the benefit just from cutting down on meat rather than eliminating it entirely. And many of the non-health benefits of a vegetarian diet are also proportional. Eating less meat means fewer animals suffer, and less damage is done to the environment. One study found that eating one less hamburger each week is like driving a typical car 320 fewer miles over a year. Raising animals using organic, humane, and grass-fed methods appears to be less environmentally damaging[17]—as well as causing less suffering.

You can also pick and choose your meats to try to minimize your impact. Lamb, beef, and pork seem to cause the most environmental damage and greenhouse gases (and honestly cheese isn't great, either). Chicken is significantly better—although chickens are small, so producing chicken inevitably involves a lot more individual animals than, say, beef. Fish is also pretty good, although the farmed varieties (like much salmon) have higher environmental impacts and sometimes more worrying quantities of mercury and other toxins.

In the end, you have to find your own middle way. Some of you are already vegetarians or may be thinking of becoming one. Good for you. Others can't imagine taking that step. Buddha's Diet doesn't require you to give up meat or cheese or any other food you enjoy. The one and only hard and fast rule is to be mindful of what you eat, and the impact it has on you and the world around you.

CHAPTER 8

Buddha's Whiskey

ALCOHOL IS A TRICKY SUBJECT. BUDDHA DIDN'T DRINK—
never, ever, not at all. In his rules for monks and even novices, "intoxicating liquors" were completely forbidden. This
is one of the few places where Buddha got really picky about
food and pretty specific about alcohol's ills, too. He outlined
these six serious dangers: "diminishing of wealth, increased
quarreling, a whole range of illnesses, ill repute, exposing
oneself, and weakening of the intellect."[1] Buddha knew even
then what a night of top-shelf margaritas could lead to. And
yes, he mentioned "exposing oneself." These spring break traditions are older than you think.

This doesn't necessarily mean *you* shouldn't drink. The Buddha became extremely celibate, too, and that doesn't mean
you have to give up sex.* But there are a few things to consider about drinking.

---

* What does it mean to be *extremely* celibate? He didn't even have sex
with himself.

First and foremost, *drinking counts*. Many alcoholic drinks are loaded with carbohydrates, which quickly become simple sugars. And alcohol itself goes straight to the mitochondria to be metabolized,[2] and so contributes to overworking these little cellular factories. Drinking outside your eating window will defeat the purpose of Buddha's Diet. You might as well eat a sundae.

Second, for lots of people, alcohol makes you hungry. Numerous studies have shown that people eat more after they have a drink.[3] You start with a beer, and next thing you know you've got a bowl of chips. You grab some cheese and crackers to go with that glass of wine. Or you reach for the ice cream. Pretty soon you're having alcohol *and* a sundae. The whole diet is out the window.

Third, alcohol really does cloud our judgment. This is probably why Buddha didn't like it. And he *really* didn't like it. He once said that if "repeatedly pursued," alcohol would lead to rebirth in hell, which is about as tough as he gets.[4]

Any diet requires you to exercise discretion. Overeating is certainly not the worst thing you can do under the influence, but it may be the most common. It's just hard to make good choices when you've had a few drinks. So even during your regularly scheduled meals, you'll want to be careful.

Finally, even for the most abstemious among us, alcohol is often part of a larger celebration. And those festivities don't necessarily end at 6 p.m. or 7 p.m. or whenever your predetermined eating window closes—at least not the good ones.

This makes it harder to stick to the diet. If that's the case for you, you might limit alcohol to only those special occasions. It's much harder to decline a glass of champagne to toast a birthday than to decline it on a regular Tuesday night. You can make these late-night celebrations your cheat day for the week. (We have a chapter on cheating coming up.)

Having said all that, there is some reason to believe moderate drinking could be healthy—at least wine and other drinks without a lot of carbs. (Beer is pretty universally agreed to be bad. Sorry.) Wine, in particular, has been shown to improve insulin sensitivity, which could counteract the metabolic stress of eating too much sugar. [5]

Be careful though. If you are having two glasses of wine at night to "unwind," it's important to think honestly about whether alcohol has become something of a crutch. Alcohol shouldn't be what you reach for to calm your nerves—just as food shouldn't be what you reach for when you've had a sad or stressful day. Buddha advocated mindfulness rather than intoxication to still our minds. He wanted us to wake up, not pass out.

There is no real consensus on how much alcohol is too much, although just about every health authority agrees you need to set limits. Each country's health department makes a different recommendation and there is a lot of variation.[6] The U.S. guideline for women, for example, is over four times higher than Finland's, and two times higher than Germany's—which are not exactly teetotaling nations.

And ironically, there's some evidence that these guidelines are entirely counterproductive anyway. In one recent study, when students were told the precise alcohol content of various beverages, about 90% of them used the information not to moderate their consumption, but to select the most alcoholic, in the hopes of getting drunk more quickly.[7] And those same researchers found that regardless of whether the students knew the national guidelines, 77% of the women and *100% of the men* said they drank "more than they personally believed was responsible."

We all have to find our own middle way. For some, that may be drinking only on special occasions. For others it will be something more—but not too much more. Special occasion or not, we recommend limiting your alcohol intake to no more than two standard drinks per week. Why two? For one thing, that seems to be the threshold at which alcohol starts to cause measurable sleep problems—and we have a whole chapter soon on the importance of sleep. Beyond one to two alcoholic beverages per week, scientists find that the more you drink, the less you sleep.[8]

And what is a "standard" drink? The official U.S. definition is 14 grams of actual alcohol—which is the amount in roughly 12 ounces of beer, 5 ounces of wine, or a single shot of harder stuff like whiskey or gin. It's not much—if you have a pint of beer or a tall glass of wine, that already counts as a bit more than one. You can have both your drinks on one night, or divide them across two. That's it.

You may find this is still too much drinking (and calories) to get to your goal. Or you may find you can imbibe more often, depending on how the weight comes off. As with everything in Buddha's Diet, you need to pay attention to how alcohol affects you and your body and adjust accordingly. But it's a good place to start. The most important thing is to make a choice and stick to it. Choose now.

What about nonalcoholic drinks? Buddha didn't have a lot to say about that. In fact, drinks are technically exempt from his no-eating-after-noon rules. Of course, he lived before refrigeration. Milk required finding a cow, and juice would have been available only when fruits were in season, and probably not in large amounts. (Making your own juice without a fancy juicer is *hard*.)

These days, some Buddhist monks in Thailand have been exploiting this liquid loophole—with disastrous effects. Researchers there found that some drinks can have as many calories as four servings of rice.[9] With so many monks drinking sugary sodas and fruit juices all afternoon, obesity and diabetes are now serious problems. Lots of studies link liquid calories to weight gain, and drinks with added sugar seem to have a direct effect on your waistline.[10] This is one place where you need to be stricter than the Buddha. Drinks *count*. Don't drink anything with calories after hours—and avoid sugary drinks any time as much as possible.

Buddha and his monks were probably drinking water most of the time—and so should you. Water is calorie-free and healthy, and staying hydrated is important. In Buddhist temples today, water is often offered as a symbol of purity, clarity, and calmness. Offer some to your body on a regular basis.

Black coffee and plain tea (black or green) have few to no calories, so you can drink these any time. The situation changes quite a bit with fancier coffee (or tea) drinks. Starbucks has somehow convinced otherwise intelligent adults that a 20-ounce milk shake is a reasonable snack. It's not. These drinks can have over 500 calories, as much as a small meal, and about half of it from sugar, which is the worst. This is a huge tax on your metabolism. Treat it as a dessert.

What about a middle ground, like a splash of milk in your coffee or a bit of honey or sugar in your tea? An ounce of milk has somewhere between 10 and 20 calories, depending on whether it's skim or whole or something in between. That's not a lot. But the time-restricted feeding experiments allowed *no calories* after hours—zilch, zero, none. All those mice got was water. We don't know how things would have turned out if they spiked the water with a little milk or sugar, so we are advocating complete metabolic rest outside your eating window. The safest approach is to have your tea or coffee plain.

The science is somewhat mixed on caffeine—some studies suggest it's good for you,[11] others not so good.[12] If you like it, there's no compelling reason not to drink it. Some people find it reduces their appetite, which might be helpful in the early days of changing your eating schedule. But if it keeps you up at night, switch to decaf. Remember that good sleep helps weight loss as well, so if caffeine is keeping you up, you may be sabotaging the diet.

Would Buddha drink diet sodas? They are filled with scary-sounding ingredients, and while scientists don't worry so much about artificial sweeteners causing cancer anymore,[13] they do seem to disrupt our metabolisms in ways we don't yet fully understand. Some studies also suggest that people who drink diet soda unconsciously compensate by overeating elsewhere,[14] so they may not be effective in cutting calories to begin with. One study of several hundred senior citizens found that those with a daily diet soda habit added a full three inches to their waistline on average over ten years, compared to less than an inch for those who abstained.[15]

The greatest concern these days is that artificial sweeteners can induce glucose intolerance, which means disrupting the body's ability to handle ordinary sugar. Because they pass through our stomachs undigested, these artificial sweeteners interact directly with all the good bacteria living in our guts. Called the intestinal microbiota, those microscopic creatures are vital to our digestive systems, and play a role in everything from obesity to diabetes. And somehow the sweeteners throw them out of whack. In one study, giving perfectly healthy volunteers the maximum recommended dose of an artificial sweetener for just *seven days* produced measurable impairment to their glucose metabolism.[16] So we suggest keeping clear of these on Buddha's Diet.

When all else fails, drink some tea. Really. You'll be amazed how many problems it can solve. We like to think of it as Buddha's whiskey.

CHAPTER 9

Cheating on the Buddha

NOT SURPRISINGLY, BUDDHA DIDN'T REALLY BELIEVE IN cheating. Several rules for monks and nuns relate to various forms of dishonesty. Monks weren't allowed to lie, of course—but that was just the beginning. Slander and gossip were also forbidden. As we mentioned before, monks weren't even supposed to shuffle food around in their bowl to make it look like they didn't have much, because that might mislead the faithful into giving more than they should. And one of the most serious rules of all forbids monks from telling women they can improve their karma by sleeping with them. It's a little sad, but even 2,500 hundred years ago, Buddha needed a special rule to keep monks from being scumbags.

But there's another side to these rules that's easy to miss in the flood of dos and don'ts. Forbidding certain behavior is only half the rule, after all. The other half is the punishment. And in many cases, there was no punishment at all.

Buddha felt these rules were important, but he also knew that everyone made mistakes. There was no point pretending otherwise. So from the very beginning, he established a simple ritual. On the day of the full moon each month, monks would assemble as a group and each one would confess the rules he'd broken since the last time they'd met. And then—unless it was one of a handful of super serious offenses—they'd move on. No shaming, no punishment. For most of the rules, acknowledging the mistake was enough.*

As in all things, Buddha believed in moderation here, finding a middle way between a rigid life obsessed with rules and a free-for-all where anything goes. So he made rules for monks. A lot of them. But he also understood that they wouldn't be able to follow all the rules all the time.

In dieting, the situation is even more complicated. It's not entirely clear that being 100% strict about your diet is even a good thing. The issue is that your body adapts over time to the food environment around it. If your body isn't getting many calories, it starts to think food is scarce and begins to conserve energy. It actually fights to prevent losing weight, assuming every pound is precious.[1] Your metabolism slows down to make what you're eating last longer, and your body releases hormones to make you hungrier to motivate you to look for more food.[2]

---

* Not for the scumbag rule, though, in case you were wondering. On that point, Buddha didn't mess around: you did it once and you were kicked out of the monkhood.

But when you're *trying* to lose weight, this is the opposite of what you want. You don't want to eke out everything you can from each calorie—you want to burn through them like there's no tomorrow. These unhelpful metabolic adaptations in response to dieting might explain why so many people hit weight-loss plateaus after a few months and can't seem to lose any more.[3]

Thankfully, there are reasons to believe cheating a bit can help.

It's hard to study cheating scientifically. If you ask people to cheat as part of a study, it's not really cheating anymore. And if you just look after the fact at what happened to dieters who followed every rule and dieters who didn't, you won't really know what caused whatever differences you find. Maybe people who stick to the letter of their diets are just different from people who don't. Maybe those sticklers live their lives differently in other ways, too.

Still, research has shown that overeating now and then can speed up our metabolism, causing us to burn more calories,[4] and can reset some of those appetite-controlling hormones.[5] This is exactly what you *do* want. There are also lots of anecdotal reports that cheating can make some diets more effective, presumably for this same reason. It's similar to the way taking an occasional break from certain medications prevents our bodies from getting habituated to them and rendering them less effective over time.

So Buddha's Diet allows you to have one "cheat day" each week, during which you let yourself eat outside your normal schedule. You don't *have* to do this—it's not an ironclad rule that you eat after hours once a week—but if it happens, it's absolutely okay. In fact, you'll likely find that a cheat day will help you succeed on Buddha's Diet, mainly because there is often something that comes up during the week that will throw off your eating schedule—a birthday, a work dinner, an evening event at your child's school. In these situations, the cheat day becomes a necessary part of accommodating the rest of your life schedule. If you have something that happens weekly—maybe Friday or Saturday night is a date night and you want to have a late dinner or some popcorn with your evening movie—that can be your cheat night. But it's also fine to have your cheat day be more sporadic, based on what the week throws at you. The important thing to remember is that the cheat *day* should not become cheat *days*. Once you're having multiple cheat days, you're not on Buddha's Diet. You can take off one day a week—but that's it.

This approach has been used by professional athletes for years. Bodybuilders who need to lose weight for competitions often use 24-hour periods of "refeeding"—where they increase their calorie intake, especially of carbohydrates—and there is evidence that this helps them avoid those metabolic adjustments that would otherwise make further weight loss very difficult.[6] Other research on ordinary, overweight men and women found those who take a break from their diets don't seem to have worse weight-loss outcomes than those who stick to them more rigidly, as long as they get back on track quickly.[7] So short bouts of cheating don't seem to hurt, and may very well help.

Buddha's Diet is designed to be a way of eating that you can stick with for the long term—a way of life, if you will. We certainly hope you haven't gone out for a late-night dinner with friends for the last time. We don't want you to skip every after-work party or family event. Buddha's Diet requires some flexibility to last—and adding a cheat day can be a form of scaffolding under the diet, supporting you and your goal.

The most important thing is never to get discouraged. If you end up eating a late-night snack once, don't let that be an excuse to give up on Buddha's Diet. Enjoy it, move on, and make doubly sure you stick to the diet the rest of the week. If you've cheated once this week, that's no reason to slide back into your old way of eating. Instead it should motivate you to double down on your schedule for the next few days. That little bit of overeating has prepped your metabolism to make the most of Buddha's Diet for the rest of the week.

CHAPTER 10

Did Buddha Do CrossFit?

YOU SHOULD EXERCISE. YOU'LL FEEL BETTER AND LIVE longer. You'll probably look better, too. You'll get better muscle tone, which most people seem to like. But exercising alone won't make you thin.

You *should* be able to lose weight by exercising and burning off all those excess calories—right? It makes sense. But for most people it just doesn't work. And when scientists have tried to prove it does work, they've almost always failed.

Why? Mostly for two reasons. First, exercise doesn't burn as many calories as you'd think. Running a brisk 10-minute mile probably takes between 80 and 150 calories, depending on your weight. That's less than half a Snickers bar—or about as much as a good-sized banana. That's it—for running *a mile*. To work off a thick slice of cheesecake, you'd have to run half a marathon.

Second, for most people, exercise makes you hungry. Your

body knows that exercise burns calories, and it's trained to eat afterward. It's called working up an appetite. You probably felt this all the time as a kid, running around outside or swimming at the pool and coming home famished. The same thing happens now when you go to the gym—if you're not careful, you'll eat more afterward than you would have anyway.

But none of this means you shouldn't exercise.

Exercise combined with a healthier diet has a lot more promise than exercise alone. And exercise has many, many other benefits—stress relief, stamina, heart and lung function, just to name a handful. And while exercise on its own won't burn away the extra pounds, it can help make your diet more effective. Many of us are emotional eaters or simply absent-minded eaters—and we have whole chapters on these topics coming up. We might eat when stressed, sad, frustrated, or angry. Maybe you've found yourself at the end of a truly awful day, crawling under your child's bed in search of hidden Halloween candy. Or you've started digging through the freezer to excavate an ancient tub of Rocky Road. When our stress level is off the charts, or when we've gotten a bit of bad news, we tell ourselves we deserve some junk. And then we feel even worse.

While there is momentary relief upon eating your snack of choice, it doesn't last. Tasty, sugary foods cause the release of dopamine deep within our brains. It's the same basic process that makes certain drugs so addictive.[1] But just like drugs, the dopamine thrill wears off fast, and over time we need more and more sweets to get the same effect.[2]

The old advice about taking a walk to clear your head actually *does* work—exercise really can help with depression and anxiety. A recent study out of Stockholm suggests that exercise prevents depression in the first place.[3] Ordinary mice get depressed when they're stressed—just like you. But the Swedish researchers found that exercising regularly breaks down this link. The stress probably still wasn't fun for the mice, but it didn't cause signs of real depression as long as they were getting regular exercise. It will help your spirits, too. You can use exercise instead of food as your relief—from sadness, from anxiety, or from boredom. As your mood improves, the emotional eating you were doing falls by the wayside.

Buddha didn't do CrossFit or any other trendy fitness regimen—unless you count yoga, which he certainly tried. But he got a lot of exercise. People picture him sitting quietly under a peaceful tree (which he did) or perched atop a lonely mountain (which he wasn't), but he actually spent much of his time walking around. In the earliest days of Buddhism, Buddha and his followers were nomadic, wandering all over India. The original words for monks and nuns—*bhikkku* and *bhikkuni*—meant "beggar," because Buddha and his followers went out on foot every morning begging for food, often for hours on end. And they usually kept moving after their meal, traveling from place to place each day without any permanent home. They only settled down during the annual monsoons, when heavy rains made travel impossible on the primitive dirt paths that passed for roads. Once the weather cleared, they were off walking again.

As the modern Vietnamese Buddhist teacher Thich Nhat Hanh explains, walking can be another form of meditation—and a very valuable one. He encourages his students to focus on their breath as they walk—and to smile. Walking in this way, he says, "is a way to remind oneself that mind and body are two aspects of the same thing."[4]

And so Buddha's walking tradition has continued to this day. If you wake up early in Bangkok, you'll still see the saffron-robed monks wandering the streets with their begging bowls. In the austere Zen monasteries of Japan, the monks don't always wander the countryside, but they perform serious physical labor—often quite demanding—in addition to their endless hours of meditation. They still quote the sixth-century abbot Baizhang admonishing that "a day without work is a day without eating."[5]

A lot of people like to do their exercise first thing in the morning, just like those mendicant monks. It helps them wake up and start the day. But how do you do this if you're not eating breakfast until 9:00 a.m. or 9:30 a.m.? Is it healthy to exercise on an empty stomach?

It may feel strange and counterintuitive at first, but exercising before you eat is perfectly natural. Before humans had figured out food storage about 10,000 years ago, everyone started the day with some strenuous hunting or gathering, and only ate after they had found food[6]. Furthermore, it turns out that exercising on an empty stomach burns 20% more fat than doing it after a meal.[7] Why? The calories exercise does consume have to come from somewhere, and if your body can't get them from breakfast, it'll take them from your thighs or belly or wherever else you might have fat to spare. So all that walking Buddha did before his first meal each morning was even more beneficial.

What kind of exercise should you do? That really depends on you, your abilities, and what you like. Do you hate the gym? No one is going to make you go. Are you bored by yoga? You don't have to do that, either. Why? Because you need to find exercise you enjoy. There's a reason new gym memberships spike in January and then plummet shortly after. The gym is not for everyone, and finding something you'll stick to is most important.

Maybe the only exercise you get right now is running after your children or taking the stairs at work. It doesn't have to be an all-or-nothing approach. Just because you didn't sweat it out for an hour on a treadmill, doesn't mean it wasn't worth doing. A study of over 50,000 adults in Texas between the ages of 18 and 100 found that running for even just five to ten minutes a day significantly reduced their risk of death, particularly from heart disease.[8] Just five to ten minutes! A study in Denmark uncovered similar results, with men and women who jogged even a little increasing their life expectancy by an average of about six years. As the researchers summarized: "Irrespective of jogging duration, pace, and frequency, the mortality was lower among joggers than non-joggers."[9]

So a ten-minute walk with the dog is better than nothing at all. Maybe you can do push-ups against the edge of the kitchen counter while the coffeemaker drips or the water boils in your kettle. Maybe you can do calf raises while you're brushing your teeth. Just start by doing *something*. It doesn't have to be training for a marathon or taking a 75-minute spin class. The worst thing you can do is resign yourself to a sedentary life because you think you could never exercise enough. Even a few minutes of exercise will leave you feeling better equipped to take on the day. Literally, every little bit helps.[10]

As in everything else in life, Buddha taught that we need to find a middle ground in exercise—not obsessed with our bodies, but not neglecting them, either. "To keep the body in good health is a duty," Buddha told his first monks, because otherwise we can't "keep our minds strong and clear."[11] That's the right way to think about exercise—a powerful path to staying healthy and sane.

CHAPTER 11

Buddha at Rest

BY NOW YOU WON'T BE SURPRISED TO LEARN WHAT BUDDHA said about sleep: he taught that we should get enough, but not too much. In one lesson, he used the analogy of a musical instrument, which is in tune when its strings are not too tight and not too loose.[1] In the same way, he wanted us to be neither too restless nor too lazy. Buddha did worry a bit about oversleeping—which he lumped in with adultery, picking fights, evil friends, hurting others, and stinginess in a list of six things in life to avoid.[2] (It's hard to disagree with any of these.) But he nevertheless thought it was important to get enough.

The Centers for Disease Control has estimated that over 35% of American adults get less than the recommended seven hours of sleep each night.[3] We've all heard of those rare geniuses like Albert Einstein who reportedly didn't need to sleep more than a few hours. Let's be honest—you're probably not one of them. We certainly aren't. For mere mortals, sleep is vital. And lack of sleep causes lots of problems. Poor sleeps disrupts our natural circadian rhythms, which are implicated in everything from cancer and heart disease to premature aging.[4] And lack of sleep is *strongly* associated with obesity.[5]

How do sleepless nights make us fat? Too little sleep seems to disrupt the hormones that control appetite and satiety,[6] with the net result that we're just more hungry the next day. One study took a group of sedentary and overweight adults and had them complete two 14-day trials at the University of Chicago. In one, the volunteers slept 5½ hours; in the other, they slept 8½. (They were monitored all day during these two-week stays to ensure they didn't nap.) All their food intake was carefully measured. Their meals didn't increase much, but the short sleepers ate over 25% more snacks. And they tended to eat at the worst times, increasing their snacking after 7 p.m. by a whopping 57%.[7] Maybe we just have more self-control when we're well rested, but another study confirmed that people who get enough sleep reported "fewer cravings for sweet and salty foods in the evenings."[8] That's a huge help on Buddha's Diet.

Short sleep is also associated with emotional eating,[9] causing us to eat even more when we're stressed. We have a whole chapter on emotional eating ("Food as Comfort, Food as Reward") because it can be such a barrier to a healthy diet. And not sleeping well and not sleeping enough make it worse.

Poor sleep also decreases our insulin sensitivity and glucose tolerance[10]—which means it makes sugar even *more* fattening than it already is. Sleep problems also reduce our energy expenditure, meaning we burn fewer calories. If we're sleeping less, shouldn't we be more active? Actually it's the opposite—sleep disruption makes us more tired, with the end result that we get less exercise the following day than we otherwise would.

It gets worse. Not only does lack of sleep often lead to obesity, but obesity also disrupts our sleep. In some cases, it can lead to sleep apnea or other sleep disorders.[11] All this creates a vicious cycle. As one researcher described it, we end up with "shortened sleep causing weight gain and weight gain causing shortened sleep."[12]

But you can turn this cycle around. Weight-loss diets appear to work better when you're getting enough sleep, in part because that lack of sleep otherwise makes us hungrier and more susceptible to binge eating.[13] Often the best predictor of whether a weight-loss program will be successful is whether the participants are getting enough sleep.[14] In one intensive weight-loss trial among 472 obese adults, those sleeping 6 to 8 hours per night were significantly more likely to meet their goal of losing at least 10 pounds in six months than those sleeping less than that.[15] Another recent study of 123 men and women in a weight-loss program found similarly that both length and quality of sleep determined how much fat participants lost.[16]

So a better night's sleep will help you lose weight and losing weight will improve your sleep. At first you may find it hard to fall asleep on an emptier stomach. But while going to bed several hours after your last meal may take some getting used to, researchers find that nighttime eating actually disrupts our sleep.[17] Over time you should find yourself sleeping better on Buddha's Diet than you did before, which will help you lose weight, which will help you sleep even better, and on and on.

Of course, getting enough sleep is one of those things like eating your vegetables and exercising regularly that you've probably been told to do all your life. And there's certainly more to it than the food component, though you will find that curbing the nighttime eating will help a great deal. So how else can we get better sleep? Buddha had some ideas about that, too.

Buddha promoted good sleep as one of the benefits of meditation. He knew, way back then, that a good night's sleep can flow from a clear head. "The peaceful one sleeps well," he explained, "having obtained peace of mind."[18] He also understood that nighttime is when we tend to get overwhelmed with our own recriminations and regret. It's when we're lying in bed at the end of the day that all our "evil actions"—what he called our "bodily, verbal, and mental misconduct"—can overcome us, "just as the shadow of a great mountain peak in the evening covers, overspreads, and envelops the earth."[19]

You probably haven't done anything truly *evil* during the day. But chances are you've had a few moments you aren't especially proud of. Or perhaps it's something out of your control that has you unsettled—a family member who's ill or an upcoming job interview. How often have you gone to bed, relieved that the bad day is finally over, only to find that all the anxiety, stress, and guilt is still right there in bed with you? The lights go out and suddenly you're wide awake, replaying the hurdles of the day or anticipating the hurdles of the next one.

Several recent studies show that basic mindfulness techniques can help improve your sleep. In one, sleep patients who meditated daily for just eight weeks increased their nightly sleep by over an hour.[20] Another study found that long-term meditators reported significantly fewer sleep complaints.[21] The researchers surmised that mindfulness meditation probably helps sleep in several ways—by relaxing your body, by clearing your mind, and by reducing your overall level of stress. They also found that practicing mindfulness impacts your body's release of cortisol—a hormone closely tied to both sleep and stress—even in novice meditators.

There's a whole chapter coming up on meditation, but even simple exercises can help you prepare for sleep.[22] Here's one: try lying on your back and relaxing every muscle in your body so that you are sinking into your bed, with only the mattress holding you up. Start at your feet and release any tension you can feel, inch by inch, until you reach the top of your head. Then watch yourself breathing in and out, in and out, and let all other thoughts drift away. Don't reach for your phone. Don't watch TV or even read a book. Don't think through everything that went wrong that day or might go wrong tomorrow. Just relax and breathe.

It may not feel natural the first time, but don't give up. Mindfulness and meditation are skills like any other. Practice makes perfect.

Another tool you can use is exercise. We discussed lots of reasons for getting exercise in the last chapter. But if you needed one more, good physical activity will also help you sleep.[23] Exercise, sleep, health, and weight all appear to be tightly related: exercise makes you healthier and sleep better, healthier people sleep better and weigh less, weighing less makes you sleep better and healthier, and so on. Improving any one of these helps you improve all of them. The same is true for reducing stress. Less stress improves sleep, curbs poor food choices, and helps keep us at a healthy weight. Then that healthy weight further reduces stress and fatigue and helps us get an even better night's sleep. And so another vicious cycle becomes a virtuous one.

Finally, we need a daily break from light in the same way we need a break from food. Our bodies are complex systems, most of which run on daily cycles, creating our natural circadian rhythm. But unlike a computer, for example, our bodies don't have a centralized clock that keeps all of these systems in sync. Instead we have multiple clocks, each of which tries to align itself with the "true" time of the outside world. Food is one way these clocks get reset—because our ancestors ate only during daylight, the arrival of food was a good signal of the start of the day, and a lack of food meant it was time to shut down for the night. But light has always been an even more reliable signal. The presence of light triggers all sorts of chain reactions in our bodies to wake us up or keep us awake—even when our eyes are closed.

So it's important to think about your light diet as well as your food diet. Just as you've learned to stop eating at a certain hour on Buddha's Diet, you also need to find times to eliminate light. Try using dimmer lighting in the parts of the house you use most in the evenings—certainly the bedroom, but also perhaps the living room or family room or other spaces you tend to hang out at the end of the day. A typical bedroom these days is illuminated at 300 to 500 lux—hundreds of times as bright as the candlelight or moonlight our ancestors lived by at night. You should also favor "warmer" bulbs with more orange light and less blue, because it's the blue light that triggers the wake-up reaction in our body.

We've talked about how our ancestors hundreds of years ago couldn't easily have prepared a midnight snack even if they wanted to. Well, they couldn't do much else at night, either. They didn't have a whole lot to do when the sun went down—and they probably slept more as a result. A group of scientists in Argentina studied the Toba/Qom indigenous group living in the largely rural northeast of the country.

As they explain, while some tribal members live near local towns, "others live in relatively isolated villages of 20 to 600 people and still rely on hunting and gathering for at least part of their subsistence."[24] The town-dwellers have access to electricity, while the others don't. Sure enough, those without electricity get nearly an hour more sleep every night. And that's compared to the members living in other very rural areas, without nearly as much access to media and technology as we have. So the full impact electricity has on *our* sleep is probably even higher.

Most of us now have no end of entertainment options to keep us occupied at all hours of the day and night, and we can work anytime by grabbing our laptop or picking up our phone. But sometimes those phones and laptops and TVs are gateways to the land of restlessness and worry.

When it's time to sleep, cut out all light—including phones, TVs, and other screens. You can even try a sleep mask if the outside light is bright, or if your sleeping partner is uncooperative. Whatever you need to do, give yourself some real darkness every day, so you get a break from light the same way you get a break from food. It's essential to create boundaries. Staying up that extra hour won't just leave you feeling sleepy the next day—it could undermine your diet and your health. As busy as he was meditating and teaching, Buddha carved out time for sleep. Just like you're choosing to stop eating at a certain hour each day, make the conscious choice to stop everything else at a sensible time, too.

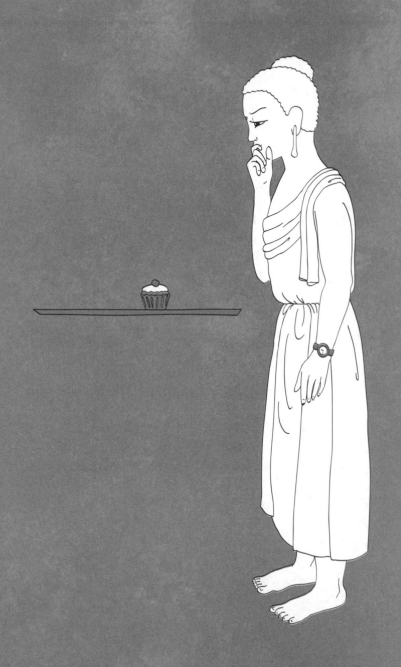

PART 3

HINDRANCES

CHAPTER 12

Food as Comfort, Food as Reward

PICTURE A LIFE IN WHICH YOUR EVERY WAKING MOMENT is spent searching for food. Your belly is distended and your limbs are emaciated like a starving child's. Your hunger is ceaseless and painful, but your throat is no wider than the eye of a needle. When you find food, you can't swallow it. Not even a bite. The hunger persists, and your search continues. Such is the fate of *pretas* in Buddhist tradition—the Hungry Ghosts.

These poor souls were reborn this way because in past lives they were driven by desire, greed, anger, and ignorance. While you might find yourself checking a few of these boxes on any given day, in Buddhism, you have to take such vices to the extreme to end up with such a tortured existence—like committing murder in a jealous rage. So no need to panic.

It's a tradition in many Asian cultures to leave offerings of food for the Hungry Ghosts. But this doesn't really help. It turns out these ghosts aren't really searching for food. Or they are, but their search is misguided. Hunger for the ghosts has nothing to do with food, and everything to do with what they did in their previous time on earth. There's plenty of food for them, but they can't eat it. Like every religious parable, there's an important lesson here: it's not food they really need.

Back here in the human realm, we still look to food to do much more than nourish our bodies and satisfy our hunger. We turn to food in times of great joy and great sadness. When something wonderful happens, we celebrate with a dinner out. We drink champagne, we eat cake, we splurge on nice meals. Food becomes part of the rejoicing. And the opposite is true, too. There's a long tradition of providing food to those who are grieving. We band together to provide meals to friends in crisis—you may, at some point in your life, have signed up on a spreadsheet or e-mail thread to bring meals to someone mourning, someone recovering, someone struggling. In times of sadness, we instinctively want to provide comfort in a tangible way. And very often, we do that with food.

Food is there for all of it—the good times and the bad. And to some extent, it makes sense. It's fun to go out and celebrate a raise, an anniversary, or a graduation. And it feels right that when people are truly suffering, the last thing they should worry about is putting together a meal. In these moments of tragedy or triumph, food is a worthy and welcome ally.

The problem comes when we use food to comfort and reward ourselves when the stakes are much, much lower. *Finally I got the kids to sleep, now I can eat those cookies I've been eyeing. That big meeting today was a mess, time for a big glass of wine.* These mundane highs and lows are challenging. But they are not worthy of great sadness or great celebration. Or, really, food.

And we know it, too. Imagine going out for dinner to celebrate fixing the washing machine. Or delivering a meal to a friend who had a bad sunburn. It sounds ridiculous. But we still give ourselves mini rewards for minor successes, and mini comforts for minor irritations—and they often involve food. We won't buy ourselves a celebratory cake, but we might well take a slice if there's some in the refrigerator. Or we might find ourselves a bag of chips or a cold beer. Each of these could easily be several hundred calories. And worse still, it's generally at the end of a long day that we find ourselves wanting this reward or comfort—the worst possible time for our bodies. Do that regularly, and it adds up fast.

There's a reason we do this, of course. Food is a natural reward. Think of Ivan Pavlov and his studies of classical conditioning in dogs—he trained them with food.[1] The comfort foods we usually turn to—the ones full of starch and sugar— are scientifically proven to improve our mood.[2] Ever hear someone refer to a particularly enticing snack as being "like crack"? Eating tasty food seems to activate the same parts of the brain as addictive drugs[3] and even cause the release of natural opiates.[4] Studies have shown that carbohydrates in particular increase serotonin release, the chemical in the body that boosts mood. The more serotonin, the better you feel. Fatty foods are the same. Brain scans of participants in a 2011 study, who were fed either a solution of fatty acids or a saline solution via a feeding tube, showed that those who got the fatty acids had less activity in the areas of the brain that controlled sadness, even after listening to "sad classical music."[5] (Yes, people actually volunteered for this study—with sad music *and* a feeding tube.)

So what's wrong with that? Better than actual crack at least, right? If food really does help with our mood, isn't that a good thing?

Yes and no. But mostly no. Remember those Hungry Ghosts? They get a bit of relief when they taste the food on their tongues. So do you, studies tell us—and you're luckier than the Hungry Ghosts because at least you can swallow your chocolate.[6] But that relief is temporary. The bad day still lingers, smothered by the brownie, or pretzels. And just like the Hungry Ghosts, you aren't *really* looking for food. What the ghosts truly want is relief from the void created by desire, greed, anger, and ignorance—yet *they keep trying to fill that empty feeling with food, even though it never works.* Sound familiar?

Not only are these self-soothing snacks not all that soothing, but when we use food to comfort and provide relief from stress, we're using it at a time when we can least afford the calories. A recent Ohio State University study of 58 healthy middle-aged women revealed that experiencing one or more stressful events the day before eating a single high-fat meal actually *slowed* their metabolism. And not just a little—enough to "add up to almost 11 pounds across a year" according to the authors.[7] Stress seems to causes the body to freak out and cling to the calories, thinking it might need them later. This may be a biological holdover from times of famine, or when we weren't all that sure when we'd spear our next woolly mammoth. Whatever we're stressed about today—whether an ill loved one, a struggling relationship, a financial burden, or a lousy job—probably won't cause us to starve tomorrow. But our bodies haven't evolved to know the difference.

And it gets worse. Overeating for any reason often leads to these same negative emotional states that then trigger more overeating. A study of both normal-weight and overweight women in Germany found that they felt sadness, shame, and anxiety after eating high-calorie foods—with the overweight women reporting the most intense emotional responses.[8] So we overeat when we're sad or stressed, then get more sad and stressed when we overeat. In between, we gain weight, which is also associated with depression and makes everything worse. It's another vicious cycle of "overeating, weight gain, and depressed mood."[9]

Luckily, there are many ways to deal with stress.[10] The healthiest approach is to take steps to address the actual cause. That may mean facing the reality of a bad relationship, or seeking out a new job, or saying no to commitments that have you stretched too thin. Social diversion—basically hanging out with friends or family—also works well. In fact, of all the ways to distract yourself, socializing seems to be the most effective.

What psychologists call "emotion-oriented coping"[11] is the most dangerous. This is when you blame yourself, daydream, fantasize, and otherwise ruminate on your miserable life. Maybe lying in bed listening to sad music. Don't do that. This often leads to emotional eating—perhaps because it just doesn't work on its own. Awfulizing rarely makes us feel better.

On the other hand, meditation and mindfulness have been shown to help significantly—a few minutes of pure silence and peace—and we'll explain all about that in a later chapter. Similarly, studies of yoga for relieving stress and anxiety are very promising,[12] and have even shown that yoga can reduce preoccupations with food for those with serious eating disorders.[13] As we already discussed, physical exercise has long been known to improve our moods, and also seems to help us fight anxiety.[14] Exposure to nature helps many people.[15] You may have to try several things before you find something that works for you. But don't let yourself use food as your cure.

What about the flip side, when we use food to reward ourselves for something good? This approach is also deeply ingrained. Parents frequently offer food (especially sweets) as a reward for good behavior—which sends a very confusing message. As one pair of researchers explained: "Parents may encourage their children to eat healthy foods, but at the same time, reward good behavior with unhealthy foods. This teaches children that some foods are good for you, but the foods that are bad for you can be earned by being good."[16] We then carry this confused and confusing philosophy with us as adults—and even impose it on our own children. In one survey of American college students, adults who rewarded themselves with food were significantly more likely to have been rewarded with food as children.[17]

But eating our rewards brings new problems. As we just discussed, these treats sometimes bring their own emotional baggage—the guilty pleasures carry a lot of guilt. If our "reward" makes us feel sad, anxious, and ashamed, it's not much of a reward, is it? This seems to be more of an issue for women than men, presumably because of the greater stigma our culture attaches to overweight women.[18] And it's worst of all for women on a diet.[19]

One of the reasons we reward ourselves is because of something called "licensing." And licensing is something we do all the time, in all kinds of environments. A study done on reusable shopping bags revealed that while people who brought their own bags bought more organic food (maybe not that surprising), *they also bought more junk food*, specifically cookies and chips. The good deed of bringing their own bag seemed to give them a license to be more indulgent in their shopping.[20] When we do something we see as virtuous, we allow ourselves more treats.

But all these rewards can easily get out of hand. Is getting your kids into bed or finishing up some work really worth rewarding yourself with an onslaught of late-night calories? Remember, this isn't about going out to celebrate an anniversary or a raise. This is about offering ourselves treats for completing the mundane tasks of every day.

Buddha taught that when we do good and virtuous things, we should do so without expectation of reward. We should do them because they are the right thing to do, not because they give us a free pass to destroy a slice of cheesecake.

You will slip up, of course, now and again. These are hard habits to break. But think carefully about just how often you are granting yourself these rewards and comforts, and see them for what they are—a temporary fix that can cause a lasting problem. And remember the lesson of the Hungry Ghosts: the unsettled self can never be sated with food.

CHAPTER 13

Food for Thought, Thought for Food

ONE OF BUDDHA'S MANY RULES FOR HIS MONKS AND nuns was that they should eat their food "with attention focused on the bowl."[1] It seems odd—maybe even a bit rude. What's wrong with a little eye contact during the meal? Maybe even some chitchat. Why treat lunch like a funeral?

It was probably Buddha's way of encouraging mindful eating.

There's been a lot of attention paid lately to mindfulness—corporations now offer mindfulness workshops to their employees, and elementary schools teach children mindfulness to help with empathy and anxiety. Mindfulness is now so popular as a strategy, a concept, a practice, that it's become a bit of a buzzword.

And it's extended to eating, too. A few experts say we

should be mindful of what we are eating, how we are eating it, and where it came from.[2] Some promise weight loss if we concentrate hard and chew our food 30 to 50 times. That's each bite—and it's next to impossible. By the time you're ready to swallow this one pulpy morsel, you've probably already forgotten what the food even was, the exact opposite of mindfulness. It's become unidentifiable goop in your mouth, smothered in saliva.

But under all this hype is something very valuable, especially as it relates to food. When we don't eat mindfully, we eat mindlessly. Two researchers from Cornell asked 139 people how many food-related decisions they made in a typical day—decisions like when, what, how much, where, and with whom they would eat.[3] Not only did they find that people were making most of these decisions unconsciously—*participants underestimated the number of decisions by over 200.* That's 200 mindless food-related decisions in just one day. And mindless eating almost always means eating poorly and too much.

So how do we practice mindful eating effectively? The first step is to recognize just what kind of mindless eating you're most likely to do. Though there are all sorts of reasons we eat mindlessly, they fall more or less into three buckets. We'll call them Meal Multitasking, Emotional Eating, and Full Not Finished.

The first type of mindless eating is something we all do now and again, fitting eating into something else we have to, or want to do. We're Meal Multitasking. Maybe you're hurrying to get somewhere and so you eat on the go, sneaking bites between stop lights. Or maybe you're on your laptop, trying to get some work done while eating your lunch. Or—something we all have done at one point or another—you're spending your evenings eating in front of the TV.

You can probably think of lots of cases of Meal Multitasking in your own life, but consider the extreme example of the movie theater. Eyes glued to the screen, we devour handful after handful of junk food, completely unaware of how much we've actually consumed until the lights come on. Next time you're leaving a movie theater, take note of the garbage around you, the popcorn knocked over, the candy boxes cast away, the lurid blue drinks tipped on their sides. It's the picture of regret—people stepping over the mess as though ashamed to be seen with their own bad choices.

One study found that moviegoers ate 45% more popcorn when it came in a large container rather than a medium-sized one.[4] Our tendency to munch mindlessly was so strong, even people who *disliked* popcorn ate 33% more when given a large! In another test, 62 women attended two 30-minute sessions, and were asked not to eat for two hours before each visit. In one session, they sat in a room with various snack foods, but were given nothing else to do. In the other session, they were offered the same snacks, but this time watched an episode of *Friends*.* In both cases they were

---

* "*The one with the red sweater,*" in case you're wondering. It was chosen because it has "no highly emotive scenes or direct references to eating." But it's still pretty good.

told to eat as much as they wanted. On average, the women ate *55% more* of their favorite snacks while they watched TV than when they just sat around for half an hour—even though they were probably more restless and bored without the show.

Of course, no one is going to give up eating movie-theater popcorn. And having a slice of pizza while watching your favorite show certainly isn't the end of the world. But if you're doing this kind of eating all the time, your lack of attention is adding pounds, plain and simple. You're far more likely to eat outside your eating window when you're doing it without thinking.

If this resonates with you, we ask you to do this: try eating without doing anything else. Not watching TV, not working, not driving, not scrolling through your Facebook feed. Just eat. You will be amazed at how different it feels. What you'll notice is that in the absence of a screen or other activity, you are forced to actually look at your food, just like Buddha asked of his monks. And when you look at your food, when you actually pay attention to the what and the when and the how much, you will make better choices. Those choices will help move you toward your goal and keep you eating less, eating better, and most important, eating only within that critical window.

Research shows that even tiny changes can have an impact. In one study, people were asked to restrict their eating at home to just their kitchen or dining room.[5] They lost weight as a result. Others were instructed that any time they thought they might eat when they weren't actually hungry, they first had to say (out loud) "I'm not hungry, but I'm going to eat this anyway." They lost even more. Yes, there will be those days when you will have to shoehorn a meal into some other activity—while you work, perhaps, or in your car. But it should not become a habit. If you've been eating so many lunches at your desk that you can shake enough crumbs from your keyboard to produce a whole sandwich, it's time for a reset.

The second type of mindless eating is Emotional Eating. We just talked about this in the last chapter, but it's worth emphasizing again. Emotional Eating is when we eat when we are happy, sad, angry, or bored. And we do this for good reasons—studies have shown that even just thinking about traditional comfort foods makes people feel less lonely, perhaps because it reminds us of our emotional bonds to others.[6] But if you're emotionally eating, you're sabotaging this diet. Emotions aren't tied to a time of day, and if anything, many of us find our poorest choices are made late in the evening as we attempt to unwind from the day's stress. You will not succeed on Buddha's Diet if you are allowing your emotions to control your eating and push you outside your window.

The third type of mindless eating is Full Not Finished. This can happen even when you are doing all the right things—eating sitting down, with a plate, not distracted, not multitasking. If you've ever said, "I ate too much," you've succumbed to Full Not Finished. When we do this, we don't even get that feel-good boost that emotional eating can provide. We just feel gross.

This usually happens because we are eating too quickly. As kids we often ate quickly because we wanted to do something else, like play with our friends. We tell our kids to "Slow down! Chew!" But as adults, we still haven't learned to do this ourselves. And because we don't slow down, we don't stop until it's too late. When our bodies have had enough to eat, they produce leptin, a hormone that tells our brains to stop looking for food.[7] But releasing this stuff, getting it to the brain, and then acting on the signal takes a bit of time. That's fine if you're foraging in the forest—you probably won't find much more before the message shows up. But in the modern world, we eat and eat and eat until at last the signal arrives in the brain and tells us to put on the brakes. By then we've had at least ten mouthfuls more than we should have. That's some of what's behind these extreme calls to chew food so many times—it slows down your eating so the brain gets a chance to catch up.

How do you know you've had enough? You don't always. In fact, we're so bad at judging how much to eat that our bodies often instead rely on external clues, like whether we've finished our plates. Just like those mindless movie-goers we talked about, research volunteers served a meal on bigger plates ate much more than those served on smaller plates.[8] Worse, they didn't even realize it—73% insisted they ate the same amount, and 19% thought they ate less! Similarly, people eating from a "bottomless" bowl of soup (refilled from a hidden tube in the table) ate almost twice as much as those eating from a normal bowl.[9]

But by slowing down, and paying attention, you'll get a much better sense of whether or not you've had enough. The goal is to eat so that you feel satisfied with what you've had, and enjoyed it, not to eat until there is no more room. Take a moment to breathe between mouthfuls. Try to notice what you're eating, how it tastes, and how it makes you feel. That signal from your stomach to your brain needs a head start, and it won't get one if you're eating too fast. If Full Not Finished is a regular part of your eating routine, you need to heed the same advice you were given as a child: *slow down.*

You don't need to eat silently, with your eyes on your plate, like the monks do—just like you don't need to stop eating immediately after noon. But Buddha's Diet asks us to pay at least some attention to our food. This mindful eating doesn't need to become an obsession. At first, you may need to remind yourself to be mindful of what you eat and drink. But with time, it becomes natural, effortless. You won't be eating on automatic pilot, just for something to do. Instead, you'll find yourself enjoying your food more fully, and noticing when you've had enough.

CHAPTER 14

Romancing the Buddha

IN MANY RESPECTS, BUDDHA'S DIET SEEMS A LOT EASIER for monks and nuns than for the rest of us. They dwell alone as solitary hermits or live with like-minded monastics following the same rules. They don't get invited to late-night birthday bashes with friends, they're not dating, and they don't have kids wanting to eat long after their own eating window has closed.

It's true. Most of us live complicated lives filled with temptations and distractions. We might need to stay late at work or attend family get-togethers that extend long into the evening. Living with or around people eating on very different schedules certainly makes Buddha's Diet more difficult. But lots of people have overcome these obstacles, and so can you.

Dating is an obvious challenge. How do you stop eating at 7:00 p.m. or 7:30 p.m. in the evening if you're meeting your date at 8:00 p.m.?

Lunches, brunches, coffee—all these are still options and perhaps more casual and relaxed than meeting for dinner, especially in the early days of dating someone new. If you've ever had a first date not go so well, you know it can be hard to wrap things up politely, except maybe by feigning fatigue—or in dire emergency, the dreaded fake phone call. A coffee or lunch date has a more natural end. Everyone expects we've got other things to do during the day, so it's no big deal to move on.

There's also no sacred law that dates have to involve eating—or drinking. What we think of as "restaurants" seem to have first appeared in Paris about 300 years ago, but couples managed to meet and fall in love for many centuries before that. If you really think about it, watching someone eat a meal isn't a particularly good way to get to know them. And while alcohol may help you relax on a first date, romantic decisions are probably best made sober.

So consider nonfood options for at least some of your dates. Go for a hike. Visit a museum. Hear some live music. Explore an interesting new neighborhood or park. All these have the advantage of not requiring you to sit staring at each other for hours, and of providing some natural material to talk about. Many people find these sorts of active dates less awkward than meals—and you can do them inside or outside your eating window.

And it's not as if you can *never* go out for a late dinner or drink on Buddha's Diet. You can use your cheat nights for dates. Some people find it helpful to stick to a rhythm for these anyway, so you can designate Friday or Saturday as your cheat day and venture out accordingly.

For some people, dating may cause other eating challenges. Studies have shown that "interpersonal stress" leads to overeating, particularly in women. Scientists have gone as far as measuring the hormones involved in appetite regulation, and they found that the one that makes you hungry (ghrelin) goes up while the one that makes you feel full (leptin) goes down when women experience interpersonal tension.[1] And what's something that can involve a lot of interpersonal tension? Dating. So be careful. Keep in mind that it may take extra effort to stick with Buddha's Diet when you're navigating relationship ups and downs.

What about the other end of the spectrum: How can you stick to Buddha's Diet if you've already got kids eating at all hours of the day or night?

It's usually possible to set up your eating window so that at least some of your meals overlap with the rest of your family's—and the easiest to align are often dinners. So if your kids eat dinner at 6 p.m., plan to eat breakfast after 9 a.m., and preferably after 9:30. That may seem tricky at first, but it's one less thing to worry about as you're rushing kids out the door. Get your kids fed and off to school, and then take your own breakfast break later in the morning.

Does it make sense to try to get your kids on Buddha's Diet? As hard as it is to study nutrition in adults, it's even harder to study in children. Controlled experiments are nearly impossible. This makes good data on kids' diets very hard to come by. A lot of what experts recommend comes from pure observational studies, or even just common sense. So if your kids are growing up healthy and fit, there's no real reason to make a change to their diet. You don't want to create unnecessary food or weight anxiety if they are doing just fine already.

Furthermore, research has shown for years that imposing eating restrictions on kids is generally counterproductive, causing an increase in their eating when not hungry, a decrease in their ability to self-regulate their diets, and ultimately weight gain.[2] One study on over 100 parents and their kids a decade ago concluded that "parental control has no impact on the child's diet" and "using food to control behavior was found to have the reverse effect."[3] More recent work confirms that restricting certain foods seems to increase kids' preference for those foods, and cause them to eat more of them when they can.[4] And all this only seems to get worse once the kids leave home.

What does seem to help kids is modeling healthy eating. One study in England surveyed over 200 teenagers living at home, and then followed up with them 12 months after they had moved out. Their results were clear: "a parent's own behavior is a far better predictor of a child's behavior after they have left home compared to parental control."[5] Or put another way: "it would seem that what parents do, rather than what they say, has the greater impact upon their children in the future."

So if your kids are already struggling with their weight, modeling a healthy, sustainable diet for yourself may be the best medicine you can provide. Buddha's Diet can help them develop good habits, like not eating out of boredom or stress and not eating late at night. Keep in mind that kids often have an even harder time than adults sticking to complicated rules around eating, and if they are eating many of their meals at school or with friends, they may have even less control over exactly what they eat. The simplicity of Buddha's Diet may well appeal to them, and will help them develop a healthy attitude towards eating they can maintain forever.

Your kids won't be interested in hearing about the eating habits of an Indian prince who lived thousands of years ago, but they will understand your simple rule of not eating after a certain time. You can explain that the kitchen is closed after a designated hour, that you're not running an all-night diner. They are free to keep eating if they want, but they are on their own. When the dishes are in the sink or the dishwasher and the table is cleared, you are done for the night. Maybe they'll make a snack for themselves or maybe they'll wait and have a bigger breakfast, but they certainly won't starve.

Sometimes navigating a diet with a spouse or partner is even more challenging than with children. Although some Buddhist traditions have relaxed the rules now, Buddha's first monks and nuns weren't allowed to marry or have any romantic attachments. They could live according to Buddha's exacting regulations on where to sleep and what to wear without having to negotiate with anyone else. But for those of us living with another adult, much of life involves negotiation. And eating is no exception.

As with kids, you should be able to plan your schedule so some meals will overlap with your partner's—although he or she may need to meet you halfway. Maybe you can push your breakfast a bit later in order to match when they eat dinner. If one or both of you needs to work late, perhaps you can meet for an early dinner, and then go back to the grind. Or try the opposite—make time to sit down for breakfast with each other in the mornings, knowing that you'll be having dinner too early to eat together in the evenings.

Of course, you can try to convince your significant other to join you on Buddha's Diet. But we recommend a *very* soft approach. Not surprisingly, "weight-teasing and other hurtful weight related comments" have been found to be extremely counterproductive.[6] Studies have shown that even "encouragement" to diet by a significant other is generally perceived as "inherently critical and negative" and is associated with the development of serious eating disorders.[7] The effects seem to be worst when it's men giving such feedback to women—but no one seems to find it very helpful.

So once again, your best bet to win over your partner may simply be modeling a healthy diet yourself. Buddhists tend to take the long view anyway and to forswear proselytizing. After all, Buddha believed we have all the time in the world—if we aren't enlightened in this lifetime, there is always another. At the same time, he taught that each life is precious, and should be lived to its fullest. Whatever you do, don't fight about food. Remember the study about appetite and interpersonal stress? People in distressed marriages have higher levels of that hunger hormone, too.[8]

Once your partner sees you looking and feeling great, they may well take the plunge on their own. Remember, too, that while not everyone is dissatisfied with their weight, many of us would like to change the types of food we're eating. Your spouse or partner may find that by following the simple rules of Buddha's Diet, they eat less junk, drink less alcohol, and sleep better. And whether they decide to try the diet or not, they'll soon be getting a healthier, happier partner—you.

CHAPTER 15

Buddha at Work

ANOTHER OBSTACLE MANY OF US FACE IN NAVIGATING Buddha's Diet is work. It's a problem of simple math: if your eating window is nine hours per day, and you're spending at least eight hours each day on the job, then chances are you'll need to do some of your eating at work. And we're including all kinds of work here. If you're a stay-at-home parent, you may be even more susceptible to poor eating choices, and your work day extends much longer than nine hours. If you do shift work at odd times, you'll have other special challenges to consider.

Eating in a healthy way on the job—any job—is not easy. As one study explained, "recent polls suggest that a third of employees felt pressure from their managers to work through lunch, with similar numbers eating lunch at their desks."[1] Half of office employees polled said they had too much work to take a real break for lunch. If you're a stay-at-home parent this may be doubly true—your schedule is dictated by your children, and they aren't known to be accommodating bosses.

One of the challenges with eating at your desk or while juggling kids at home is that you are probably eating mindlessly. At the office, you're on your computer or phone, multitasking various things. At home, you may be trying to squeeze in lunch between a child's checkup, a stop at the park, a few errands, and a nap—though probably not for you. We've already had a whole chapter on the pitfalls of multitasking your food; we just don't make good food choices when we aren't paying attention. And we won't know when to stop if we're eating on autopilot. You're much more likely to have a healthy lunch if you give it a bit of focus.

A real lunch break will do much more than help you eat right. Just as our metabolisms need a break from food, our minds need a break from work. We need time to recover from work-related stress—at the end of the day, but if possible also in the middle. Some researchers believe that the lack of time for this recovery is a bigger health concern than the sheer quantity of stress itself.[2]

A study of 103 administrative employees at a large North American university found that those who relaxed during lunch experienced less fatigue at the end of the day.[3] Interestingly, it wasn't just working through lunch that left employees exhausted—socializing at lunch often had similar effects. Sometimes we need a break not just from work, but from our coworkers.

If you're a stay-at-home parent, this may be the part of the chapter where you're shaking your head in dismay, knowing a leisurely lunch is a laughable concept. Maybe your only break from your diminutive "coworkers" is when you lock yourself in the bathroom. But there's still good reason to make your best efforts to carve out a few minutes for a real, healthy lunch. A 2011 study of new parents found that young adult mothers consumed both more sugary drinks and more saturated fats than nonmothers.[4] (The nonmothers ate more healthy vegetables, too.) Perhaps that doesn't seem surprising—it's tough to take care of yourself when you're so engrossed in taking care of your kids. But there are other things you can do to help support yourself throughout your work day such that your children don't sabotage your health. It may mean you'll eat during your child's nap, giving your food at least 15 minutes of your attention. Or if you aren't hungry then (or their napping days are over), you can use a few minutes the night before to give some thought to what you can make or pack for the next day's running around. Whatever you can do when you have a bit of quiet (notice we say a *bit*—we're parents, too) will help prevent those bad choices when you're stressed, busy, and tired the rest of the day.

The important takeaway, no matter your job, is to recognize when you are most vulnerable. You may have figured out that to succeed on Buddha's Diet, you must be mindful of these high-risk times. At work, we're in danger of making bad choices because we are stressed, time-crunched, overwhelmed, or simply not paying attention. That's true whether you reluctantly find yourself in Chuck E. Cheese's with your kids or trapped at a desk facing a deadline.

For those in an office, there is also lots of evidence that bringing some mindfulness to your job will help your company as well as yourself. Several studies have shown that mindfulness can improve employee performance[5] and reduce staff turnover.[6] It even seems to improve creativity.[7] So taking some time to recharge and recenter during the day is likely to help your work in the long run. (And if you're home parenting, you'll be calmer, more mindful, and less likely to lose it with your kids.)

When you're eating at work, try to have your meals away from your desk and without holding your phone. Try to take a real break. You aren't shortchanging your job, since the evidence shows you'll be more productive and less stressed when you get back. Consider making breakfast a midmorning break, even if it's just 15 minutes. Either bring your breakfast with you or find a cafe where you can buy something healthy, and just eat.

If at all possible, make room for an even longer break at lunch. You can certainly eat with your coworkers if you'd like, but pay attention to whether this is stressful or relaxing. (We've certainly found ourselves eating at our desk as an excuse to avoid socializing at times.) If you're having lunch with your kids, it's probably a bit of both and can turn on a dime. Now and then try taking a lunchtime walk if you can.

A study in Australia found that a short walk during lunch improved enthusiasm and relaxation and reduced nervousness and overall stress.[8] This can be as easy as choosing somewhere a little farther away to eat rather than just down the hall or around the block. Best of all is if you can actually get to a park or any sort of nature[9]—but for many of us working in cities, that may be too much to ask.

What if your job requires you to entertain clients in the evenings or otherwise eat late meals with customers or colleagues? If it's just a matter of drinks after work, you can try the old teetotaler's trick of soda water and lime—a zero-calorie drink that looks a lot like a gin and tonic. But if you absolutely have to eat at night, you still have a couple options. If it's a very occasional obligation, you can use these nights as your cheat days and simply try to keep them to no more than once a week.

If these late-night dinners are going to be more regular occurrences, then you may need to shift to a later eating window. If your eating day can't end until 8 p.m., then it can't start until 11 a.m. It's not an ideal schedule—you may find it tough to get through the morning with just black coffee or tea, and eating so late in the evening is probably less good for your body than a more natural rhythm that follows the sun. But nothing is as bad as eating around the clock, so by all means don't let the requirements of your job stop you from trying Buddha's Diet. No diet works unless you can actually do it. Find an eating window you can follow and stick to it.

Working at home—whether with kids or in some other capacity—has its own potential pitfalls. Not only are you always on call, but the temptation to snack can be very high when you're always near your own kitchen. Staying disciplined and making good food choices when your day doesn't follow the rhythm of an office can be tough. You'll need extra vigilance and planning, but it can be done.

Shift work—jobs that take place largely outside normal daylight working hours—make healthy diet (and sleep) even more difficult. Many studies link shift work to obesity and other metabolic problems,[10] as well as increased stress and poorer sleep[11] (which themselves also contribute to weight issues). Shift workers tend to have less healthy diets, and to gain more weight over time.

Of course, it's very hard to limit your eating to a 9-hour window during the day if you are working only at night—maybe even impossible. As we discussed back in chapter 4, "Buddha's Diet," shift workers may just have to make the best of a bad situation. Again, the worst diet is one where you eat at all hours of the day and night—so even if eating only at night isn't ideal, it will almost certainly be an improvement.

Another way our eating can get out of sync at work is jet lag. If your job requires you to travel a lot, you'll have to juggle Buddha's Diet while changing time zones. The best approach is to get yourself eating on the "new" time as quickly as possible. If you can avoid it, don't eat right before your flight, and fast until you arrive at your destination. Then eat a large meal at the appropriate time for your new time zone, and stick to your Buddha's Diet schedule on local time.

Fortunately, there's some evidence this can actually help you adjust more quickly. The basic symptoms of jet lag—drowsiness and wakefulness at all the wrong times—come from our bodies' attempts to match our internal clocks to the expected light-dark cycle. But it seems when there's no food during the "day," our bodies will naturally shift to stay awake at night. So even if you find yourself waking up at 3 a.m., don't order room service or hit the minibar. If you restrict yourself to eating during the local daytime, you'll help reset your clocks more quickly.[12]

As an aside, many of us experience a mini "jet lag" every weekend by allowing ourselves to sleep later than we do during the week. In one survey, a third of adults experienced two hours of this social jet lag each weekend, while two thirds had at least one hour, and this appeared to be a contributing factor to obesity.[13] In another study, sleeping in on weekends was linked not only to greater insulin resistance and a higher body mass index, but also to lowered levels of "good" cholesterol.[14] So please watch those lazy Sundays. Whatever your working schedule, you should keep a consistent eating window on your days off—and try to get enough sleep on weekdays so that you don't need extra on the weekends.

As we'll discuss later in the book, Buddha considered "right livelihood" to be one of the eight essential components of his path to enlightenment. Jobs are an integral part of life for most adults. Whether it's inside or outside the home, nine-to-five or odd hours, sticking to Buddha's Diet at work will be essential to your success.

It all comes back to focusing on your food, giving it the attention and time it deserves. Your work has importance for lots of reasons. But whatever the value of work, food shouldn't become an afterthought. Spend the time to make it the main thought, even if for a short while.

CHAPTER 16

Waste or Waist?

AS CHILDREN, MANY OF US WERE TOLD TO CLEAN OUR plates. Sometimes this was linked to dessert. *You can't have cake until you finish your dinner.* Sometimes it was linked to preventing hunger too soon in the future. *If you don't eat now, you'll be hungry later.* Sometimes it was linked to money. *You ordered that expensive dish from the menu, now you have to finish it.* And sometimes it was linked to waste, and maybe a bit of guilt. *In other countries, poor children don't have enough to eat, and here you are wasting food.*

People hate to waste food. But we do it. A lot. In North America, approximately 42% of all food is wasted, which works out to 1,520 calories worth per person.[1] That means every day each person wastes almost as much food as it would take to feed *another* person that day. All this waste clogs our landfills and greatly increases methane emissions, a powerful greenhouse gas contributing to global warming. And it leads to lots of wasted water, fertilizer, and cropland.

In many respects, we've become more responsible about food. We worry about food safety. We buy and eat more organic, local, and humanely raised food. But we're still throwing plenty of that feel-good food in the trash. And while plenty of food waste occurs during production, packaging, and distribution well before it gets to your shopping cart, over 60% happens after purchase.[2]

As we mentioned earlier, you probably grew up being told not to waste food. In a study of 122 American adults back in 2003, *over 80%* recalled being told to clean their plates after every meal.[3] Depending on your age and where you grew up, you or your parents or your parents' parents may even have seen real food shortages during wartime, when wasting food was treated as an affront to your country. If you were to go back in time and tell your great-great-grandparents that today there would be so much food around that obesity is an epidemic and we throw food *out* on a regular basis, they'd probably be simultaneously incredulous and appalled.

But here we are.

The first step in reducing waste and eating only what you need is changing your mind-set. And you will need to waste some food now in order to *stop* wasting food later. You'll see why in a moment.

This process will be challenging—remember that you are probably trying to undo years of ingrained ideas about wasted food. What we ask you to do is at each meal, once you are full and feel like you've had enough, carefully consider whether the rest of that food is better off in the trash or in your body. In other words, you have a choice to make: You can *use* the garbage can or you can *be* the garbage can.

The knee-jerk reaction may be that this food you aren't hungry for is better off in your body, where it can provide nutrition and energy and not end up in a landfill. But remember, you're full. And more than likely, you aren't planning to crawl into a cave later to hibernate through the winter. You'll be eating *again* in a few hours. You not only don't need the food, you may even find yourself feeling lousy if you finish it off. Also, what you may feel compelled to finish could have zero nutritional value.

So again, do you really want to be the garbage can?

Being the garbage can means you eat more than you want to. It means extra calories, extra weight, and quite possibly the related diseases that can come with that weight. It also means you are ignoring the signals telling your brain you are full. Your body says, *please don't eat that.* But you ignore it, you spite it. You tell it, *yes, I know you don't want me to eat anymore, but too bad, I can't bear to waste it.*

What if instead, you chose the right garbage can, the *actual* garbage can—or better yet, the compost bin, which at least lets the leftovers nourish the earth? Are you wasting food? Absolutely. But you won't help anyone by eating it. If you genuinely feel that you will eat it tomorrow, or for your next meal, by all means save it. If you're at a restaurant, take it to go. But think carefully about this, too. Sometimes taking food to go just means you're going to discover the mystery box in the back of the fridge a week later and toss it then—wasting both the food and the extra packaging. You know yourself better than anyone else. Be honest. Are you going to eat it later? No? Then compost it now.

Forcing ourselves to finish our plates means giving someone else control over how much we eat. It could be the chef at the restaurant or the packager of the ingredients or even a partner or friend, if you're lucky enough to have someone else do the cooking—but it's not you or your body. Think about the last time you went out for pasta. Like most of us, you probably finished your plate of penne or ravioli or whatever you ordered. Now what are the chances that the cook knew precisely how much you wanted to eat and served you exactly that much? Basically zero. Maybe you ate at a homestyle restaurant that heaps the plates full like an Italian grandmother, or maybe it was a fussy little place that serves tiny portions that look more like artwork, but either way the amount of food you got had little to do with how much you needed, let alone how much you wanted.

Much of the time, we don't even know how much we're eating. Many studies have shown how susceptible we are to visual cues about how much to eat. In one, diners who used a larger (10-inch) plate served themselves 50% more at an all-you-can-eat Chinese buffet than diners who used a smaller (8-inch) one. But they didn't just take more and eat more—they wasted 135% more, too.[4] The same researchers conducted another study where they randomly assigned people to two buffets—one with 9-inch plates and one with 11-inch plates—and told them they only had time to serve themselves once. In this case, the diners with larger plates took *90% more*.

These biases are deeply ingrained. Most of the volunteers in these studies vehemently denied that factors like plate size had anything to do with how much they ate. The good news is that this means most people using smaller plates will eat less and waste less and not even notice. The best way to waste less food is to serve yourself less food—and one way to serve less food is to use smaller plates. This isn't always easy. Two scientists studied vintage dinnerware for sale on eBay and found that American plates have gotten 23% *bigger* since 1900.[5] By looking at depictions of the Last Supper, they found that this trend goes back at least a thousand years, with plate size increasing about 69% since the year 1000![6] To switch to small plates, you'll need to buck this trend.

If you have children, you will also need to be careful about a few more things. First, kids are even more susceptible to these visual cues than adults—so the bigger the bowl or plate, the more food they'll take.[7] Sometimes that's good—we want our kids to eat—but it can also lead to more waste. So as parents, it's important not to let yourself start eating their meal, too. When it's time to clear the dishes, it's tempting to eat those last few bites of whatever's leftover rather than "wasting" the food you may have worked hard to cook—

even when you're plenty full yourself. You have to stop that. Don't worry about finishing off your own plate—and definitely don't finish anyone else's, either.

Something else to note about children is that we are always modeling for them. Remember that signal that tells us when to stop eating? Kids have it, too—even toddlers.[8] Encouraging them to continue eating (either with rewards like desserts or with threats of punishment) will eventually lead them to ignore that signal entirely.[9] Pressuring children to clean their plate will only lead to more waste and bigger waists when they get older.

Those living alone have their own obstacles. A study in the United Kingdom found that four-person households generated less than half the food waste per person as people living alone.[10] You might expect the opposite—that those big families with kids would be wasting tons of food. But the reason is likely that cooking just one portion is sometimes difficult, and raw ingredients are often sold in larger quantities. This can make overeating a real temptation for single people.

No one wants to waste food. Much of our desire not to waste is well-meaning. Once you can curb your tendency to overeat this excess, you'll get a better sense of how much you are wasting, which will in turn inform the amount you buy. All this will lead to less waste *without* overeating.

In the meantime, it's okay to throw things out. Just learn from it. Next time, buy less. Serve less. Order less. In a way, it's a return to those old values about food and waste. Before this modern age of cheap food, people wasted less because they had less to waste. As a World War II poster implored: "A clear plate means a clear conscience. Don't take more than you can eat."

The most obvious place you'll struggle with the impact of this new mentality is at the grocery store. These stores have evolved over time. Generations ago people shopped at multiple places for their groceries. They stopped at the butcher for their meat, the bakery for their bread. And they generally did this every day, buying just as much as they needed for the next few meals. But now we want a one-stop shop. We're busy. The new norm is to shop at places like Costco or Big Lots where we can get our groceries and our televisions at once—and the bigger the better, for both. Volume buying is encouraged even in regular grocery stores. You may have to recondition yourself to resist the myriad "buy one, get one free" promotions so prevalent these days. Do you need two? If it gets wasted, the fact that it's free isn't anything to feel good about.

It's important when you buy groceries to be honest about your intentions. They may be good (*I'm going to cook every night this week!*) but then you find that by midweek all the optimism behind that organic three-pack of romaine lettuce has been crushed by the business of work or school or simply *life*. A week later, you're not sure it's good anymore. A couple days after that, you're sure it's not. So into the trash it goes. Be realistic about your cooking plans, not aspirational. Maybe allow yourself to shop more often, buying less each time. You probably have a very good sense for what you're likely to cook today, and a pretty good sense for tomorrow. But most of our cooking predictions get haphazard beyond that. An extra trip to the grocery store is probably a lot less wasteful than a discarded meal or two worth of food.

As you adjust to buying less, you'll toss less, too. At first you may find yourself grocery shopping too often as you figure out how much you're actually eating. But soon you'll find a happy medium. You'll eat less. You'll waste less.

You'll have to readjust at restaurants, too. The custom now is for the waitstaff to encourage appetizers, and to leave bread on the table. Before we've even decided on what we want to eat, we're already eating—maybe even overeating. And unless you really like leftovers, portions are often far too big. It's fine to order an appetizer and eat only that. Often they are just as filling as an entrée. Or eat as the Spanish do, with a few smaller *tapas*-style plates. Or split an entrée between two.

Most important, remember that overeating is just another way of wasting. Yes, hundreds of millions of people suffer from malnutrition around the world.[11] But your overeating won't feed them. That extra food was already wasted back when you bought, cooked, or served yourself too much to begin with. Forcing yourself to eat it now is tackling the problem far too late. Overeating doesn't solve the waste problem. And it creates potential health problems for yourself or your family that will only lead to other sorts of waste down the road—wasted time, wasted money, even wasted lives.

CHAPTER 17

Hunger or Habit

MANY OF US HAVE A VERY LOW TOLERANCE FOR HUNGER. We tend to think of eating as something we *have* to do, not *want* to do—more like breathing than, say, shopping. And yes, of course, we do need to eat to survive. But we tend to exploit this fact, by including all kinds of eating urges in the *need* category. We exaggerate our hunger, using hyperbole when we are even slightly peckish. How often have you claimed you were "starving" when it was just a few hours since your last meal? Or, how many times have you heard someone say they were about to pass out when service at a restaurant was slow or their meal was otherwise slightly delayed? If we were all truly so desperate for food, wouldn't the streets of America be strewn with unconscious, emaciated bodies?

The truth is, often we aren't even hungry at all when we eat. We're eating more out of habit than hunger. And even when we *are* hungry, we usually eat more food than we need or should—because it tastes good, or because we're used to big portions, or even just because it's there.

You may worry that you'll feel hungry on Buddha's Diet. It's true that in the early days, you may feel some occasional hunger pangs. This is likely because you used to eat later in the evening, and you haven't adjusted your daytime eating to compensate yet. And while it may seem ridiculous to think we don't know when we're hungry, we often confuse hunger with something else. Much of the time we eat because we *think* we're hungry, when, in fact, we're just looking for a distraction—from stress, from boredom, from sadness. So when you're tempted to eat off schedule, take a moment to notice how you're really feeling. Here's a good rule of thumb: if you're bored and hungry, stressed and hungry, or sad and hungry, you're probably just bored, stressed, or sad. The hungry part is something you've trained yourself to tack on, because you've found eating to be a useful distraction in the past. But it's not a *healthy* distraction.

Hunger is often habit in disguise. Your daily routine developed through a long history of training your body to eat at certain times or in certain situations. The same way Pavlov's dogs thought they were hungry when he rang his bell, you're probably conditioned to feel hungry when you start your evening rituals, whether that's coming home from a long day at work or collapsing on the couch after the kids are in bed. But the good news is that you can train yourself not to feel hungry, too. Pavlov's dogs could have been trained to do just about anything. They didn't need to eat when they heard his bell any more than you need that bag of popcorn when you watch TV.

Habits and routine are powerful, but they can be upended. *New York Times* reporter Charles Duhigg explains in his book *The Power of Habit* [1] that habits are formed in three steps, which together form a "habit loop:"

> First, there is a *cue*, a trigger that tells our brains to go into automatic mode and which habit to use. Then there is the *routine*, which can be physical or mental or emotional. Finally, there is a *reward*, which helps your brain figure out if this particular loop is worth remembering. [2]

There's nothing inherently wrong with habits. They save us lots of time and energy. If you had to consciously remember to brush your teeth every day, you'd probably forget half the time—which wouldn't be good for anybody. Instead, you have a cue (like walking into the bathroom after you wake up) and a routine (the actual brushing) and a reward (perhaps that nice clean feeling in your mouth).

Notice that there's nothing in the tooth-brushing loop about avoiding cavities or freshening your breath. Developing cavities takes too long to function as a reward—our brain needs a signal right away for the loop to take hold, and for better or worse most of us can't really smell our own breath. So while these habit loops generally start with some larger, loftier goal, they exist somewhat independently of our grand schemes. If a new study came out today proving that brushing teeth was completely unnecessary, you'd probably still brush yours the next morning. Once the habit is formed, it takes on a life of its own, regardless of the original motivation.

Luckily, research shows that good eating habits can be just as strong as bad ones, so these habit loops can work in your favor.[3] The first step is to identify that initial goal. Let's say you typically sit in front of the TV at the end of the day and have a snack. Why? Maybe you're trying to relax—but there's nothing intrinsically relaxing about pretzels or chips. There's no reason you can't replace that bad habit with something else, a kind of rewiring, so that now you connect watching TV with something healthier. Maybe you always brew yourself a cup of tea and take that with you to the couch instead. Or maybe you use the TV time to get your laundry folded. Not as fun as eating a bowl of ice cream, but way more productive and not even slightly fattening.

Or you can create a new trigger. Maybe every night after you've done the dishes, you give yourself some time for goofing off on Facebook or reading a magazine or a good book. The cue is finishing with the kitchen, the routine is the browsing or reading, and the reward is that same sense of calm and relaxation at the end of a busy day—but without the calories. Do this enough times and it will become automatic. You may not even think about the junk food after a while.

Duhigg himself gives the example of snacking at work. What's the real goal there? Probably not actual hunger. Is it just a way to interrupt your boredom? If so, "you can easily find another release," he explains, "such as taking a quick walk or giving yourself three minutes on the Internet" which provides yourself "the same release without adding to your waistline."[4] (We assume he's just kidding about the three-minutes part—but try to keep it under thirty.)

With all these things, the key is repetition. No one creates a new habit in one try—or even two or three. As Dr. John Arden describes in his book *Rewire Your Brain*, at first habits take substantial focus and effort. This engages your brain in the process. But after a while, your brain learns the pattern and reorganizes itself to make this behavior increasingly automatic. As he explains, eventually "practice will make it effortless."[5]

When breaking old habits, it's often helpful to look for ways to change the surroundings that are linked to that habit or behavior. If you don't see your usual cues, you won't fall into your usual routine. There's a reason doctors encourage smokers to try quitting on vacation—your environment is different and your routine is different. It's as if your brain is temporarily rewired, opening the door to more permanent change. Whereas you might have smoked while having a break at work, now you're visiting a museum or lounging on a beach, cues you don't associate with your daily cigarette. Retailers have known about this for decades. A UCLA study way back in 1984 found households undergoing "status changes"—big things like moving, marriage, childbirth, or divorce—are much more likely to change their brand preferences.[6] Marketers have figured out how to use this little trick to their advantage. A woman suddenly buying prenatal vitamins may signal a new baby on the way, and that enormous life change is a perfect time to introduce other new brands and products.[7] To put it simply, change offers an opportunity for new habits.

You're not going to be able to go on vacation every time you want to break a habit, and we don't recommend getting pregnant as a way to shake up your routine. But as you embark on Buddha's Diet, you may want to avoid situations and surroundings that are associated with your old eating clock. If you always snacked in bed while watching TV, maybe you should switch to watching somewhere else. And it's okay to politely decline going out to a late dinner with friends like you used to. Arrange a lunch or a weekend hike with them instead. Maybe explain what you're trying to accomplish—good friends are also supportive friends (and statistically speaking, most of your friends probably wish they could change their own diets as well). Soon enough you'll figure out how to make this all work, with earlier dinners and occasional cheat days. Eventually you may find that your old cues have lost their power, and you'll even be fine watching other people eat after your own eating day is done. But by changing up the things you normally do, you'll find that habit loop of round-the-clock eating will quickly fade.

Of course, there may be times when you are really, truly

hungry. First, know that there's no reason you need to give in to hunger pangs. You aren't going to starve. You probably don't live your life like Prince Siddhartha's early years, indulging your every whim and desire. If you feel a little tired in the middle of the day, you don't rush off to bed then and there. If someone tells you about a great TV show at work, you don't quit and start watching right away. You don't necessarily buy *every* pair of shoes that catches your fancy. Yet somehow we've taught ourselves that hunger is different. When it comes to food, we're all living like spoiled princes. If we feel even a hint of hunger, we grab a snack without a second thought.

But there's no reason to let hunger call all the shots. You can notice you're hungry and not start eating the same way you notice you're tired without jumping straight into bed. Try doing something else—*anything* else. Instead of eating as a distraction, find yourself a distraction from eating.

If you're getting hungry regularly on Buddha's Diet, you may need to think about what you're eating. Remember that proteins and fats are more filling than sugars and carbohydrates. As we discussed in "What to Eat," though Buddha's Diet is really about the *when* of eating and not the *what*, choosing the right *what* helps with the *when*. You'll find that some foods leave you hungrier than others. High-fiber carbs like whole-wheat breads and pastas keep you feeling full longer than those made from white flour. Highly processed foods, on the other hand, are designed to keep you eating.

And this may go without saying, but surrounding yourself with tempting food at night won't make things any easier. Don't do your grocery shopping when you're hungry. Don't hang out at a restaurant or bar and expect not to eat—at least not until your new eating habits have become very deeply ingrained.

Even with all this, there will be times when you feel hungry, just like there will be times when you're sad or lonely. And that's okay. Buddha taught that there are no *bad* feelings really—just feelings. Painful or pleasant, they all pass. Cravings—whether for food or companionship or even shoes—are part of life. Sometimes they don't feel good. But the answer isn't to get rid of them, because you can't. The answer is to accept them, decide what to do with them, and move on.

You may not fully control your hunger, but it doesn't control you, either. Not anymore.

CHAPTER 18

Keeping Your Balance

THE TROUBLE WITH MOST DIETS IS THAT THEY ARE DESIGNED to be temporary. We tell people we are going "on" a diet, knowing full well we'll be going "off" it soon enough. So it's not surprising that losing weight and keeping it off is hard. *Really* hard. Most people who lose weight on a diet eventually gain it back.[1]

To avoid this sort of weight cycling, it's important to think of Buddha's Diet as a permanent way of eating—a lifelong lifestyle—not a temporary fix. You don't go "off" it after a few months. Our bodies were never meant to eat at all hours. Once you've adjusted to this more natural daily rhythm, we don't want you to go back. And honestly, you won't want to, either—nonstop eating will start to feel unnatural and strange. Compared to the varied and extreme diets out there with strict rules about dairy or wheat or meat—not to mention the juice fasts, the pricey herbal supplements, and the diets that claim there's some undiscovered trick or exotic tropical berry for losing all that weight—our experience is that Buddha's Diet is a lot easier to sustain.

Even though long-term weight loss is challenging, there are plenty of people who are successful for extended periods of time. Studies of the National Weight Control Registry—a database that tracks over 10,000 individuals who have lost weight and *kept it off*—reveal that there are some common threads among those who've nailed it. The first is that most of these people had some sort of "triggering event."[2] For a few, this is a medical issue—anything from sleep apnea or back pain to varicose veins or aching legs. For others, especially women, it's an emotional trigger, such as (and this is an actual quote from a study on triggers): "my husband left me and my lawyer told me it was because I was fat."

We hope you haven't experienced any of these—and we'll assume that lawyer has been reborn as a slug, or will be soon. But whatever prompted you to try Buddha's Diet in the first place, keep that same trigger in mind as the pounds come off and you move into the maintenance phase. And if you haven't had the classic "wake-up call," don't wait for it. Keep yourself and your diet healthy right now. Don't let your weight force your hand.

What else do those who succeed in keeping weight off have in common? Well, they exercise, which is probably no surprise. Exercise in conjunction with weight loss is always a bonus. You should be exercising already for all the reasons we talked about previously. And it seems even more important in weight maintenance by counteracting some of your body's natural tendencies to regain lost weight.[3]

A few other things stand out among the weight-loss winners: 78% of successful registrants eat breakfast every day. So that adage about it being the most important meal of the day may be especially true for those trying to keep weight off—perhaps because eating early helps prevent people from eating late, which is, of course, perfect for Buddha's Diet. Also 62% watch less than 10 hours of TV a week—which makes sense. What do we know happens when we are watching TV or movies? Mindless eating. Cut down your screen time and you'll likely cut calories.

Finally, 75% weigh themselves at least once a week. Other studies confirm that weekly is about right when you're trying to maintain your weight. Put another way, the best advice seems to be to "self-weigh at least weekly to prevent weight gain and daily for weight loss."[4]

All these patterns fit nicely within Buddha's Diet. You'll do less of that mindless eating once you've cut time from your eating clock. You'll keep weighing yourself regularly. And because you aren't going to be eating late at night, you'll want to have a good breakfast in the morning that won't leave you vulnerable to bad snacking choices later in the day.

To some extent, time is on your side. The National Weight Control Registry also shows that your chances of keeping the weight off improve with every year of success. One survey found that individuals who had maintained their weight for two years reduced their risk of regaining by 50%.[5]

What happens if you find yourself tipping the balance the other way, and you're losing too much? If you are just starting out on Buddha's Diet, this may be hard to believe, but it is possible to lose too much weight. Seriously. It happens. It happened to us at some point. If you're diligent about your eating schedule, you will ultimately hit your weight goal—and maybe even drop below it. So what do you do then?

The most important thing to remember is that weight loss is not a game where the lowest score wins. Lower isn't always better. Being underweight poses real health risks, just as obesity does.[6]

On the other hand, you don't want to backslide into your old habits, either. As we said at the start of this chapter, this isn't a diet you ever go "off" completely. Remember those poor mice? The ones who ate whatever they wanted, whenever they wanted, gained weight—a lot of weight. And it didn't take long. In a few months, they were obese. You don't want that to happen to you. You don't want to be back where you started.

Instead, as Buddha would suggest, you have to find a middle ground. You can try adding an hour back to your eating schedule, so you're eating in a 10-hour window again, like you were in Step 3 of Buddha's Diet. For some, that seems to be a good balancing point, where you neither lose nor gain weight. You can also try a bit more cheating. In those mouse experiments, mice who cheated two days a week didn't seem to gain weight—although they didn't lose weight, either. So you can try adding one more cheat day to your weekly routine.

But don't let 10 hours of eating drift unconsciously to 11 or 12 and then all the way to 16 or 18. Don't let 2 days of cheating become 5 and then 7. If you find yourself slipping into old habits, and find the unwanted pounds returning, don't beat yourself up. Just dial it back again. Return to the full Buddha's Diet for another month to get on track, and then try again to find the right equilibrium for maintenance.

You've probably heard the saying you can never be too rich or too thin. In our experience, neither of those is true. And Buddha agreed. He lived as a wealthy prince and as an emaciated ascetic, and rejected both those extremes. He found his middle way. You'll find yours.

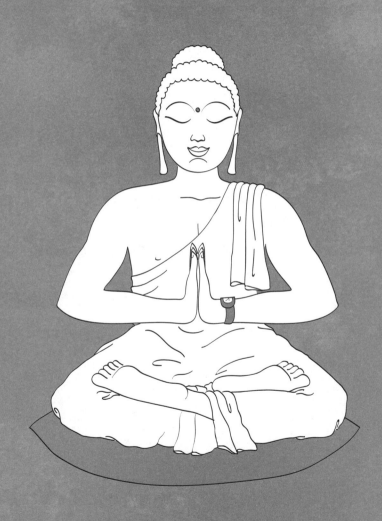

PERFECTIONS

The Wisdom of Saying Grace

MANY CULTURES AND RELIGIONS PRACTICE SOME KIND OF ritual of expressing gratitude before eating a meal. In English we usually call this "saying grace." Most Christian denominations use a variation of the traditional Catholic blessing: "Bless us, O Lord, and these, Thy gifts, which we are about to receive from Thy bounty." American Zen Buddhist communities typically recite a brief passage that begins, "We reflect on the effort that brought us this food and consider how it comes to us. We reflect on our virtue and practice, and whether we are worthy of this offering."

A common element here is an acknowledgment of food as a gift or offering for which we should be thankful. Many people are hungry and unable to enjoy a meal. Perhaps we, too, have experienced real hunger. Before digging ravenously

166 ❁ BUDDHA'S DIET

into the plate before us, we take a moment to reflect on our good fortune.

We encourage this on Buddha's Diet. You don't need to say any formal prayer, but consider pausing for at least a moment of reflection. Think about what you are about to eat. Think about why.

Establishing this tiny ritual will help you prevent mindless, reflexive eating. We've already talked about all the benefits of bringing mindfulness to the table, and this is a way to help yourself do that. Look at what's on your plate. As the Zen chant suggests, reflect for just a moment on how that food came to you. Appreciate the small miracle of having enough to eat right now.

Thinking more deeply about the origin of our food can help us make better choices in how we eat. This may be why people who visit farmers' markets start to eat more fruits and vegetables,[1] as do people who participate in community garden programs.[2] Of course, other people just end up with a crisper full of rotting vegetables—the cold compost of good intentions—and a belly full of the usual junk. Our goal is not to engage in aspirational shopping, but rather to force ourselves out of our usual routine, to stop eating so mindlessly. Frequenting these venues is another way to help us pay more attention to how and what we eat. And when we pay more attention, we make better choices. Arranging our lives to support and encourage better choices is what Buddha's Diet is all about.

Several studies have found that people who report being more religious or spiritual have a healthier diet.[3] A study in Thailand found that adults with "Buddhist values" were better able to control their diabetes through healthy eating.[4] This pattern even holds true for kids. One study of several thousand teenagers around Minneapolis found that "students who reported that spiritual or religious beliefs affected their decisions about a range of health behaviors, including eating habits, were more likely to report greater intakes of fruits and vegetables."[5]

Perhaps some would say those religious people are being guided to health by a higher power. But it seems more likely that they are simply being more thoughtful, making more conscious choices about their health and their diet. The enemy here is not atheism—many Buddhists are atheists, and Buddha himself was perhaps best described as agnostic. In one famous lecture, he criticizes teachers who claim to know God as being like a procession of blind men: "the first one does not see, the middle one does not see, and the last one does not see."[6] He doesn't deny the existence of God, but wants us to focus on our own experience in the here and now.

Once again, the real enemy is mindlessness. Those teenagers who described themselves as religious may simply have been a bit more thoughtful about their lives and life choices. Their faith may have led them to be a little more present. That is how we all should be.

The traditional Zen blessing before meals continues by

stating, "We regard it as essential to keep the mind free from excesses such as greed. We regard this food as good medicine to sustain our life." This is also important to remember. Hunger is natural and healthy. Greed is not. We are eating to nourish our bodies, not to distract ourselves from our problems or reward ourselves for our accomplishments. Eating should not be an escape.

You don't need to be religious to be on Buddha's Diet. You certainly don't have to be Buddhist. Studies have shown that the benefits of mindfulness are independent of how religious or spiritual you are. A survey of over a thousand adults in the United States and Canada found that nonreligious people were just as "moral" as religious ones—they just felt less guilty than religious people when they slipped up.[7] In another recent study, children around the world were asked to share stickers with others kids in school who didn't have any. Those who were raised religiously acted less generously than their nonreligious peers[8]—although to be fair, the authors admitted they didn't have enough Buddhists in their sample to say anything specifically about them.

So you don't need to pray before you eat. But take a moment to reflect. Be thankful. Whether any specific religious entity is thanked is up to you. You might be thankful to the countless farm workers, the factories, the processing plants, the grocery store stockists and checkout clerks, all of whom brought your food to the table. If you grew your own lettuce for your salad, maybe you're thankful for your own hard work, or the friends and family who helped (that part may be wishful thinking). Maybe you're grateful for the sun, the rain, the soil, and all the rest. Maybe you ordered a pizza and you're just truly thankful for the delivery driver who showed up and saved you from cooking. Or maybe money is tight right now and what you're eating isn't even that great—but at least you have something.

Anytime we eat, there is something to be grateful for. The Zen chant concludes, "For the sake of enlightenment we now receive this food." Pausing before we eat gives us one more chance to be mindful, to pay attention. Let eating become part of your practice. Take this opportunity not just to fill up, but to wake up.

CHAPTER 20

Meditation for Your Body

INCREDIBLE CLAIMS HAVE BEEN MADE FOR THE POWER of meditation. Some are a bit outlandish—like that you can levitate into the air or stop breathing completely or survive for weeks without food or drink. There are even reports of monks who can generate enough "psychic heat" to dry wet bedsheets wrapped around them with just the warmth of their skin. But while certain meditation techniques do seem to raise body temperature a few degrees,[1] and we'll talk about some other interesting biological effects in a moment, most of the truly far-fetched promises about meditation are seriously unlikely. In any case, we don't expect you to dry laundry with your mind—as useful as that might be.

But we do think meditation will help you. And it's really not that hard. We'll get to that in a bit, too.

Most people associate Buddhism with meditation, and for good reason. After Buddha became frustrated with ascetic life and abandoned his small company of holy men, he sat down under a quiet tree in the forest to meditate, vowing not to move until he had found enlightenment.[2] And find it, he did. From that moment on, meditation has been central to Buddhist life. Buddha went on to give countless lectures on various meditation techniques that are still studied today, and the tree where he first sat has become a pilgrimage spot for Buddhists worldwide. For many people, Buddhism *is* meditation. Everything else is window dressing.

This is an oversimplification. Not all Buddhists are meditators, just as not all Buddhists are vegetarians. Particularly in Asian countries, many Buddhists visit temples on festival days and keep an altar or shrine in their home, yet may never have meditated in their lives. But in the West, meditation is often what first draws newcomers to Buddhism, and many of the largest Buddhist organizations here are dedicated to meditation instruction.

Buddha prescribed meditation for a very specific purpose: to help us realize enlightenment. And enlightenment is not a strange mystical transformation. Enlightenment is a very basic and concrete state of mind. Enlightenment means awakening. To be enlightened is to be truly, completely awake. Back when Buddha first described the foundations of mindfulness meditation to his monks, he told them that if they just followed his instructions for seven years, they would be guaranteed enlightenment. Guaranteed! But then he corrected himself—maybe it would only take six years, five years, four years, three years, or two years. Then he decided it might take less than a year—maybe just seven months, six months, five months, four months, three months, or even one month. Finally, he settled on seven days. If they practiced mindfulness meditation diligently for seven days, that might be enough.[3] Even Buddha knew when to ease up.

What does enlightenment feel like? We all know what it means to be awake, and we all know what it means to be asleep. And most of us have had some experiences in the middle, where we're half-asleep or half-awake. Maybe it's the few minutes before we doze off at night, or the seemingly endless hours when we're daydreaming on a plane or lying at the beach.

Think of these states of mind on a spectrum. On one end is unconsciousness and sleep. Then comes those moments of half-sleep and daydreaming. Then comes our ordinary experience of waking life. And now imagine that we extend this scale just a little bit further, say a half step beyond our usual "awake," to a point where we're fully aware, fully mindful of everything around us. That's enlightenment:

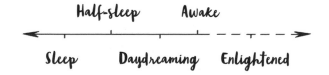

How does meditation help us get enlightened? What's the connection between meditation and the mindfulness we discussed in "Food for Thought, Thought for Food?" And what does any of it have to do with dieting?

Buddha didn't teach meditation to help anybody lose weight. He believed that meditation would help us all live a happy and awakened life—what he called "the attainment of the true way," or ultimate Nirvana.[4] And he had a very specific theory for how it could do this. Buddha taught that meditation helps us reduce what he called "cravings."

In his first lecture after his awakening, Buddha taught that the cause of all suffering sprang from *upādāna*, a Pali word usually translated as "desire" or "craving." In other words, we suffer because we *want* something. Being happy means being content, being satisfied with what we have and with the way the universe is right now. And meditation helps us let go of cravings and find that contentment and peace.

Cravings, of course, are a problem for dieters, too. We've all had the experience of a seemingly irresistible urge to eat something we know we shouldn't, or to eat too much, or to eat when we should be doing something else. Meditation helps. A group of researchers at McGill University in Montreal got 196 chocolate lovers to volunteer for an experiment. First, they were given some basic mindfulness training. For example, when they found themselves having chocolate cravings, they were told to "label them as 'just thoughts' and then imagine distancing themselves from their cravings"[5]—in much the same way we learn to let go of whatever thoughts or feelings arise during a meditation session. After this two-week training phase, participants were brought into a room and given some chocolate and told to unwrap and hold it but not eat it. Then the chocolate was taken away. The researchers found that this mindfulness training worked: volunteers who got the mindfulness training reported significantly less chocolate craving after this test than the others experienced.

Meditation seems to help with dieting in other ways, too. Because mindfulness meditation asks us to observe our feelings but not become attached to them, it teaches what psychologists call "disidentification"—the process of separating ourselves from our own thoughts.[6] This can help us avoid negative coping strategies such as emotional eating. As one scientific review summarized, "mindfulness training provides a promising approach for weight loss and weight maintenance" because it "provides individuals with skills that allow them to mitigate maladaptive eating behaviors and develop positive relationships with food."[7] It also seems to help us tolerate the discomfort associated with changing our eating habits. As a result, several recent studies have shown that mindfulness training alone can lead to weight loss.[8]

And not just weight loss. Another review concludes: "Meditators reported significantly higher levels of mindfulness, self-compassion and overall sense of well-being, and significantly lower levels of psychological symptoms, rumination, thought suppression, fear of emotion, and difficulties with emotion regulation," and that "mindfulness is positively associated with a variety of indicators of psychological health."[9] Or as Buddha put it, meditation is the path "for the surmounting of sorrow" and "the disappearance of pain and grief."[10]

How can meditation do all this? Scientists have studied the effects of meditation on the brain and body for decades now.[11] Meditation appears to make us more relaxed, and lower our blood pressure and heart rate. It even seems to transform our basic brain structure in ways that improve attention and our ability to regulate emotions. At least 21 studies have been completed on how meditation alters our neurobiology, documenting effects on many distinct brain regions.[12]

People who haven't tried meditation often think it's complicated or difficult, but despite the bewildering array of meditation techniques out there, meditation is fundamentally quite simple. In the Zen tradition, meditation is often called "just sitting" and is intended to be literally that—simply sitting still without any other plan or goal in the world.

You don't need fancy equipment or extensive training to meditate. Once you've found a quiet place to sit, here are the basic instructions the famous scholar and former monk Stephen Batchelor gives in his classic book, *Buddhism without Beliefs:* "Make sure the back is unsupported and upright, but not tense. Check to see if there are any points of tension in the body: the shoulders, the neck, around the eyes.

Relax them. Take three long, slow, deep breaths. Then let the breathing resume its own rhythm, without interference or control."[13]

See, it's not difficult. Try following these steps:

- **SIT COMFORTABLY:** The traditional posture is to sit cross-legged on a cushion on the floor, but that isn't essential. You can meditate kneeling or sitting in a chair if that's more comfortable. But sit up straight rather than slouching. If you're on a chair, don't let yourself lean back. Couches are generally not so good.

- **SET A TIMER:** Stick with sitting until your time is up. You can buy specialty meditation timers, and several apps for your phone are available with nice pleasing chimes at the end. But any timer will do.

- **FOCUS ON YOUR BREATH:** Why do we focus on our breaths? You don't have to, and some prefer to focus on a word or phrase, while still others attempt to empty their minds completely, "thinking of nonthinking" as the Zen masters used to say. But most people find the breath a good, solid place to start. It's like a natural metronome, helping you keep time with your body. If you could sense your own heartbeat, that might be even better. But most of us can't.

- **NARRATE YOUR BREATHING:** Buddha suggested that as you inhale, you say to yourself, "I am breathing in." Then as you exhale, say to yourself, "I am breathing out." If you notice yourself taking a short breath, say, "I am breathing in short." If you notice yourself taking a long breath, say, "I am breathing in long." Whatever happens, stay with your breathing. Be aware of each and every breath.[14]

- **EXPAND YOUR FOCUS:** As you get more comfortable with this breath meditation, expand your mindfulness further. Try to be aware of your whole body as you sit. Change your internal monologue a bit. As you inhale, say: "I breathe in experiencing the whole body." As you exhale, say: "I breathe out experiencing the whole body." Pay attention to all your experiences, but don't judge them. If you have pain in your back or your knees (which you might at first), notice the sensation, but don't let it distract you from your breath. If you find yourself impatiently waiting for the timer to ring, that's okay, too. Don't beat yourself up. Let that feeling come and go. Sit through it.

Start with a modest goal for sitting: 5 minutes. The first few times you may find this feels impossibly long, but it isn't. Your mind will undoubtedly wander, and you'll notice you haven't thought about your breath for a while. Don't worry. When you realize you've stopped focusing on your breath, just come back to it. Again, no judgement. This happens to all of us—even Buddha probably struggled at first. Return to your body and breath. Feel yourself inhale and exhale again. Relax.

Once you can sit this way for 5 minutes comfortably, try 10, then 15. You can stop at 15 if you'd like, or continue up to 30. The nice thing about short periods is that they are that much easier to schedule—no matter how busy you are, you can almost always squeeze in 15 minutes. But some people find they get to a level of calm in 30 minutes beyond what they find in 15. Experiment a bit for yourself and see how it feels.

Buddhists often talk about meditation as a "practice," and this is meant literally. In a fully awakened life, we would be mindful of all things, at all times. But that's hard. Our lives are full of distractions. So use meditation as a bit of a shortcut, almost a cheat. It's the opposite of multitasking. We cut away as many of the distractions as we can to make it that much easier to fully concentrate. It's like studying at the library rather than in your dorm room. It still takes work to do homework even in a quiet setting, but it's much easier when we're away from the distractions of friends and music and television and all that. And there is good evidence that this approach works, that practicing mindfulness through meditation makes it easier to stay mindful throughout the day.[15]

We can't promise enlightenment in a week, and sitting still for a few minutes each day won't necessarily fix a broken relationship or a bad job. Deadlines at work won't be magically extended, and a dwindling checking account won't spontaneously grow. But meditation will better equip you to deal with all these problems by helping you develop a calm center to return to when you feel yourself becoming overwhelmed or making bad decisions—whether about your diet or about anything else in your life.

CHAPTER 21

Defiling the Temple

WE ARE OFTEN AT ODDS WITH OUR BODIES. THEY BETRAY us in small and big ways. They get sore, they get sick, they age. At times, our genes mutate and fight against us, causing disease. Some of this is chance, some genetics, some diet and habit. But one way or the other, our bodies can feel like a foreign enemy. Even Buddha ventured awfully close to body-hate sometimes. When his students got too full of themselves, Buddha liked to remind them that their bodies were filled with "excrement, bile, phlegm, pus, blood, sweat, fat" and other nasty stuff.[1] (Really, that wasn't even the whole list.)

We expect a great deal from our physical selves, and for the most part our bodies deliver, doing remarkable things in the process. They carry children and run marathons and sometimes even save the lives of others. It was Buddha's body that let him meditate and teach and his students' bodies that let them find him and learn.

But we are also tough on our bodies. By now it's not news to you that most of us eat poorly and too much and too often. We eat junk, which is the equivalent of tossing trash into our bodies. You could say we are cruel to our bodies, expecting that they will still perform, still work, even after this mistreatment. We know this is bad—we may even regret our choices as we are still chewing. But study after study has shown that when it comes to diet, our bad habits are stronger than our good intentions.[2]

So why do we do it? Well, for all the reasons we've talked about—everything from using food to soothe, to being too busy. Sometimes we play little tricks on ourselves about all this, too: *I'll get in shape in the New Year. I'll stop smoking at my next birthday. I'll eat better tomorrow.* We figure we have time to change. Compounding this is the fact that it's not always easy to correlate our bad choices with poor health. You may even have a relative who smoked a pack a day, ate whatever he wanted, and lived to be 95. It happens.

Still, the science tells us that bad choices will catch up with most of us. Maybe not for a few years, but eventually. Yes, you may be one of the lucky ones who dodges the disease bullets. But the odds are not in your favor.

The paradox of all this is that while we are pretty cavalier with our health, we spend a lot of time and energy worrying about what we look like on the outside. So much of the diet industry is predicated on the idea that we look, well, bad. Of course, some of this is couched in health, but vanity is a strong force and we are often motivated by how we appear on the outside, not what is happening within. Would we still wear sunscreen if there was no risk of skin cancer, but without it the sun still aged our skin? We might.

The media is filled with examples of this body hatred. How else to explain the extreme photoshopping prevalent in just about every glossy magazine? Celebrities who do not fit an incredibly narrow version of beauty are eviscerated online. It's hard not to extend these unrealistic and superficial expectations to ourselves—if famous, beautiful, successful people are mocked for how they look, surely the rest of us should be hiding under a bridge. And the results are clear: about 90% of American women report being dissatisfied with their bodies.[3]

Though the most egregious examples of body scrutiny often come from the media, plenty of it happens at home and may be quite subtle. Parents might complain about how they themselves look—maybe they struggle with their weight or are themselves chasing ever-changing diet fads—and that message is passed to their child. A recent study found that even some four-year-old girls expressed a desire to be thinner—and that this was most likely in girls whose mothers were dieting.[4] That's *four-year-olds*. "Am I also fat?" they must be wondering. Another study found that by age 13, fully a third of girls were "upset/distressed about weight and shape."[5]

All this attention to thinness can be dangerous, even fatal—and the prevalence of eating disorders in our youth, especially teen girls, is proof of this. The extreme desire to be thin is at times the stuff of dark humor. Dr. Glenn A. Gaesser, director of the Healthy Lifestyles Research Center at Arizona State University writes, "Over half of the females age 12–18 studied would prefer to be run over by a truck than to be fat." *Run over by a truck.*[6]*

It's no surprise that our obesity epidemic, coupled with this hyperfocus on appearance, has given rise to the particularly cruel and unhelpful trend of fat shaming. In addition to the emotional distress and discrimination to the recipient, it also doesn't cause anyone to lose any actual weight.[7] Even if it is well intentioned, it generally backfires. In a study of over 6,000 adults in Florida, overweight individuals who experienced some form of weight discrimination were much more likely to become fully obese.[8]

Even if you haven't felt the pain of outside comments about your weight, you may well be fat shaming yourself, feeling embarrassed when you look in the mirror or hopeless and frustrated when you try on clothes. You might think this would lead to weight loss—that being shamed, either by others or yourself, would somehow be the kick in the pants you need. But there doesn't seem to be any evidence to support that. Yes, some people, realizing they can no longer button their jeans may make the decision to lose weight on their own. But hating your body, or even being overly critical will not actually help you on Buddha's Diet. Or any diet.

* The figure must be 100% for a small car

And though it may be somewhat unrealistic to hope for this, losing weight should be motivated more by health, not by what you will look like.

It may seem counterintuitive, but you must love your body before you try to change it. Why? Because this shift in thinking causes better choices. There is evidence that even very small amounts of weight loss can cause positive shifts in our body image.[9] It's as if even this little progress helps us see that our bodies are not our enemies. And then this positive attitude makes it easier to lose weight, and to keep it off.[10] Improvements in our body image help us curb emotional eating, too.[11] As you start to like your body again, you start to take better care of it in times of stress.

There's a famous quote from St. Paul's letter to the Corinthians that our bodies are temples. Think about that. If your body is a temple, shouldn't it be treated well—revered and appreciated? Why on earth are we defiling it every day of the week?

This mind-set will take practice. But ask yourself if you would go to a beautiful church or temple, or a national monument or park . . . and *litter*. Would you stand at the edge of the Grand Canyon and toss your trash into it? We're guessing not. But that's in essence what you're doing so much of the day. You are littering, defiling, and dismissing the very house, the very temple, that enables you to breathe. It's a body that does a lot of work on your behalf. You should repay it more kindly.

Think about all the things you're thankful for, all the things that your body has done and continues to do for you. Maybe it has carried babies, or healed itself after a bad accident. Maybe it climbs mountains and grabs small children as they dart into the street. Every day your body does something remarkable.

As we just described in the last chapter, Buddha taught his disciples to meditate on their body, to *experience* their body—their *whole* body—with each breath. This is the only body we have. It won't last forever. Everything we accomplish in this life—whether it's cooking a meal, hugging a friend, or finding enlightenment—we have to do through the one body we have.

As the great Japanese Zen master Eihei Dogen said, "The living body of this one day is a living body to revere."[12] You have one lifetime right now, full of gifts and experiences. It's your body that makes those gifts and experiences possible. Try to remember times you were overwhelmingly grateful for the way your body performed and consider how you can best repay It. It's not that you can never eat junk food again. You can. But treat your body like a good friend. You will find that you will be more motivated to give it better food and the free-for-all style of eating whatever, whenever will begin to melt away.

CHAPTER 22

Living Like a Buddha

BUDDHA WASN'T A DIET GURU. HE WASN'T TALKING ABOUT
mindfulness to help people lose weight, or get in shape, or
reduce stress. He wanted us to aim much higher than that.
He preached what he felt was an entirely new path based
on his newfound "middle way," which he said "gives rise to
vision, which gives rise to knowledge, which leads to peace,
to direct knowledge, to enlightenment," and ultimately to
Nirvana. He wouldn't be content with us shedding pounds.
He wanted us to shed greed, hate, and delusion.

Many Buddhists are happy to see mindfulness find such
broad acceptance in the secular world today. As one monk
and Buddhist scholar wrote, "if psychotherapists can draw
upon Buddhist mindfulness practice to help people overcome anxiety and distress, their work is most commend-
able."[1] But others have been skeptical, and even hostile to
separating mindfulness from Buddha's other teachings. One

cynical observer notes that "there is considerable enthusiasm for mindfulness these days, as long as it does not threaten to make us wise."[2] These critics argue that mindfulness can't really be understood without the original context of everything else Buddha taught.[3]

So what was the original context?

Buddha talked about mindfulness in the very first lecture after his awakening. He spoke to a small group of wandering ascetics who had gathered in a deer park outside the village of Sarnath in northeastern India. Right away his main focus was on his middle way between the "unbeneficial" extremes of self-mortification and pure sensual pleasure.[4] He mentioned mindfulness, too, but it was just one piece of an Eightfold Path that all needed to be practiced together.[5] There were seven others. We needed to practice what he called "right mindfulness" for sure. But we also needed right view, right intention, right speech, right action, right livelihood, right effort and, right concentration. Mindfulness actually came toward the end, sandwiched between effort and concentration.

If these eight seem like a lot to remember, it is. Buddha had various ways of summarizing the Eightfold Path, like combining the items into the three broad categories of wisdom (right view and intention), ethics (right speech, action, and livelihood), and meditation (right effort, mindfulness, and concentration).[6] But there's no getting around the fact that it's basically everything. How you speak, how you act, how you work—it all matters. It's not just what you do when you're meditating. And it's not just being mindful. It's everything.

Why should you do all this? Not because Buddha said so. And certainly not because we're telling you to. Buddha wasn't relaying the commandments of any god or supreme being. He was sharing a discovery he had made about how to relieve suffering, what he described as a natural law.[7] It's a bit like Newton discovering gravity. Two objects don't attract each other in relation to their mass because anyone decreed it—they just *do*, because that's the way the universe works. Gravity was there before Newton, and it would still be here if he had never described it. Buddha felt the same way about his Eightfold Path. When we "speak or act with a peaceful mind," he explained, "happiness follows."[8] It just does.

So you should do the "right" thing because that's what reduces suffering in the world. All the things we know are wrong—lying, cheating, stealing, killing—they all cause suffering. And Buddha even took this a step further. It's not just that acting immorally causes suffering—it's that an act becomes immoral *because* it causes suffering.

But don't take his word for it—try it yourself. Don't try killing, of course. But how about lying? We've all tried that already. How did it turn out? Probably not so great. And not just lying to other people—how about lying to yourself? We've all tried that, too. It's a disaster. It might feel good at first, but in the long run, it causes suffering.

This is what Buddhists mean by *karma*, by the way. Karma is Buddha's word for this natural law of cause and effect. The Dalai Lama explains it this way: "If you act well, things will be good, and if you act badly, things will be bad."[9]

Buddha did go into more specifics. As we mentioned early on, he had over two hundred detailed rules for monks and nuns. And he covered the basics for laypeople, too: no killing, stealing, lying, or sexual misconduct—he didn't define this last one, but assumed we'd know it when we saw it.[10]

But these rules just scratch the surface. For Buddha, living "right" means living in ways that reduce suffering—either for yourself or for someone else. All the time. It's a tall order, and it means thinking through everything we do. So "right speech," for example, doesn't just mean saying things that are true—although that's part of it. We should also say only what is necessary, and what is kind.

That's really what Buddhism boils down to, thinking about the consequences of our actions and always choosing the ones that reduce suffering. That's why the Dalai Lama himself has said, "My true religion is Kindness."[11]

And does it work? Can we really relieve suffering in ourselves and others?

Yes and no. When something painful happens to us, we don't just feel the immediate pain—we also have feelings *about* the pain, like sadness, anger, or regret. So we have two unpleasant feelings—a physical one and a mental one. Buddha described this as like being struck by two arrows.[12] The first arrow we can't avoid—pain *hurts*, whether we want it to or not. But the second arrow is our own choice.

Buddhist practice is about avoiding these second arrows—not shooting them and not receiving them. Maybe you have to give bad news to a friend or offer honest criticism to a coworker. It may hurt the person you're telling, like that first arrow. But we can say even painful words with kindness. We don't have to fire a second arrow with the way we speak.

It's not always easy to be kind. And none of us is kind all the time. But kindness matters.

Keep in mind that this kindness also applies to yourself. You are a sentient being, worthy of compassion. Buddha's path isn't intended to be easy. Some advanced students spend long hours every day in meditation, and that's physically and mentally difficult even for experienced practitioners. But it should never be brutal. It's all about that middle way. Don't let yourself off the hook by taking shortcuts. But don't beat yourself up if you falter now and then.

Zen master Eihei Dogen once wrote: "To study the Buddha way is to study the self."[13] This is exactly what Buddha himself did during his years as a wandering ascetic—he studied himself and tried to figure out which practices worked for him and which didn't. Buddha's Diet asks you to do the same thing. In a sense, you'll become your body's own data scientist, observing yourself as you eat to see what works for you and what doesn't. And the same applies to the rest of life—it may take some trial and error to learn which actions cause suffering and which relieve it. But you can't do this if you're not paying attention. This is the essence of Buddha's teachings—to pay attention to all our actions and their consequences.

The very next line Master Dogen wrote is in some ways even more interesting: "To study the self is to forget the self." Because at some point all this paying attention becomes second nature. The Dalai Lama isn't kind because he wants to be. He's kind because he has to be—because he's always paying attention to his actions and their consequences. It's easy to step on a bug or snail if you aren't looking where you're going. It's much harder if you see it first.

In time our speech naturally becomes right speech, because we pay attention to the consequences of our words. Our livelihoods becomes right livelihoods, because we pay attention to how our work affects everyone around us. And so on. Even our eating becomes right eating, because we naturally pay attention to when and what we eat, and how this impacts our bodies and perhaps the planet. Mindfulness becomes second nature.

In other words, we wake up.

CHAPTER 23

Not Living Like a Buddha

THERE ARE A FEW THINGS WE HAVEN'T TOLD YOU ABOUT
the Buddha. Things that aren't so great. But we think you
should know. And we'd rather you heard it from us.

When Siddhartha left home to seek his enlightenment, he
wasn't single. He was twenty-nine and had already gotten
married. Just a few days before he left, he and his wife had
had a son. But this had not filled him with domestic bliss.
He named his son Rahula, which is usually translated as "fet-
ter" or "impediment."[1] More colloquially, we might say "ball
and chain." Think about that. This wasn't Siddhartha grum-
bling with his friends about his wife and kid holding him
back—he *named his son* ball and chain.

Then he left them. He snuck away one night without
warning. Something about family life felt incompatible with
his great quest for truth. They say he crept in and took one
last look at the baby—*his* baby—before he disappeared. He

probably thought about staying, but he didn't. And it's not clear that he said anything at all to his devoted wife—who, remember, *had just given birth* that same week. But what could he say? *It's not you, it's me?* That probably didn't sound very convincing even two thousand years ago.

In other words, before he became the Awakened One, the Enlightened One, the Great Sage of India, the World-Honored One—before all that, Buddha was kind of a jerk.

This is one of the important lessons of Buddhism. Although the message got a bit muddled in later retellings, Buddha was not a god. He was not superhuman. He wasn't perfect. He made mistakes, just like all of us. And not just small mistakes, either. He made some really, really big ones.

In the end, Buddha's family forgave him. His wife even became one of the first Buddhist nuns. At first Buddha would only accept men as followers, but he eventually relented, acknowledging his earlier refusal as yet another mistake. Their son, Rahula, was ordained, too. Both are said to have found enlightenment following Buddha's path.

Buddha himself never forgot his imperfections. He never claimed to be better than he was. In his final speech, he told his monks that everything changes, nothing lasts forever, and they should always adapt his teachings as needed. Nothing was cast in stone. And in the centuries since, Buddhists have taken him at his word. When the teachings spread to colder climates like China, the monks and nuns stopped wearing the loose, flowing robes the Buddha insisted on in tropical

India and adopted something more practical—basically gray pajamas, with lots of layers. Once Buddhism reached Japan, several sects even dropped the requirement that monks and nuns remain celibate and allowed them to marry. Here in the West, many Buddhist groups have moved even further toward complete equality of men and women—something the Buddha didn't seem to think possible in his lifetime— and now give full recognition of same-sex unions, both for laypeople and the ordained.

Not all Buddhist monks follow the original eating rules these days, either. In many countries, monks now eat dinner in the evening—though usually a small, simple dish. At a temple here in San Francisco, the tradition is to serve only leftovers, so they aren't cooking a full meal in the afternoon.

Keep this in mind. Things change. We try things out and learn from our mistakes. What works for one person in one time and place isn't going to work for everyone else. Life is an experiment. You have to keep experimenting.

Buddha's dying words were, "Work hard and find your own salvation." And that still sounds about right.

CHAPTER 24

Beyond

YOU NOW KNOW ALL THE FUNDAMENTALS OF BUDDHA'S
Diet. Hopefully you're on it already and enjoying the changes
in your body and your life. So what's next? If you're interested in exploring further some of the topics we've covered
in this book, you might consider the following possibilities.

BOOKS ON BUDDHA AND BUDDHISM

1. *Buddha* by Karen Armstrong. This is the best modern
   retelling of Buddha's life. Armstrong is not herself a
   Buddhist, and brings a fresh perspective to the story that
   makes her book instantly accessible.

2. *Teachings of the Buddha* by Jack Kornfield and Gil Fronsdal. As we explained in the introduction, the original
   Buddhist scriptures are long. And not just Harry Potter

long—*long* long. Thousands and thousands of pages. Thankfully, Kornfield and Fronsdal—both Buddhist teachers themselves—have collected many of Buddha's most enlightening words into this beautiful little book.

3. *Buddhism without Beliefs* by Stephen Batchelor. Batchelor's goal is to free Buddhist teachings from sectarian distinctions and create a new vision of Buddhism for the modern world. If you're the sort of person who has little patience for anything overly "spiritual," this is the best book for you.

BOOKS ON BUDDHISM AND MEDITATION

Each branch of Buddhism has its own distinct beliefs and practices—and its own unique feel. Three of them (Zen, Theravada, and Tibetan) have gained particular prominence here in the West, so if you decide to purse Buddhism on your own, it will likely be though one of these three styles. These books can help you get started:

1. *Zen Mind, Beginner's Mind* by Shunryu Suzuki, the Japanese master who founded the San Francisco Zen Center in the 1960s. His style is very simple and direct—he is the most prominent proponent of "just sitting," without a lot of rigmarole or fuss.

2. *Mindfulness in Plain English* by the Burmese master

Bhante Gunaratana. The oldest school of Buddhism still practiced is Theravada, and this is a great introduction to their "insight" style of meditation. Insight meditation can get a bit more technical than Zen, so this book has more detail and explanation.

3. *How to Practice: The Way to a Meaningful Life,* by His Holiness the Dalai Lama introduces not just Tibetan meditation but much of the rest of Tibetan Buddhism.

OTHER TOOLS

One of the advantages of Buddha's Diet is that it doesn't require a lot of equipment or paraphernalia. But a few things can help:

1. SCALE: We recommend you invest in a good scale—and we love the networked ones that share your weight with your phone.
2. FITNESS/HEALTH APPS: There are a number of good fitness apps that allow you to track your weight over time, so you don't get hung up on any one measurement.
3. COMPOST BIN: A nice compost bin that's easy to clean is a great investment. It can even be something that works indoors, and maybe fits under your sink if you don't have much space. Remember that you don't want to be the garbage can (or the compost bin) when you're already full. Reread "Waste or Waist?" if you need a refresher on this.

And really, that's about it. There are, of course, many fitness and health books out there, and certainly a vast library of books about Buddhism. These are simply some initial suggestions. One of Buddha's lessons is that you already have everything you need. The next step is up to you.

Acknowledgments

SOME LOVELY PEOPLE HELPED MAKE THIS BOOK POSSIBLE. First, we are grateful to our families who offered encouragement and support. Our thanks also go to our friends Dr. Matthew Baggott, who first introduced us to the scientific literature on time-restricted diets, and Jennifer Wright, who shared her own insights into diet and nutrition. Thanks to Dr. Mark Mattson for reading an early draft of our book and providing us his sage advice. We're grateful to Laura Dail, our agent, who championed the book from its earliest beginnings as a 5-page draft, and Jennifer Kasius, our editor at Running Press, who shepherded it into the form you hold now. Their excitement has been contagious.

This book would not have been possible without Dr. Satchin Panda's groundbreaking research at the Salk Institute. Not only were his findings invaluable, but the kindness and generosity he extended to us were above and beyond. And finally we thank Buddha, who figured all this out a long time ago, and inspired us each along the way.

Endnotes

INTRODUCTION

1. Bhikku Nanamoli, *The Life of the Buddha*, (Onalaska, WA: BPS Pariyatti Editions, 1992), 18.

2. Karen Armstrong, *Buddha*, (New York, NY: Penguin Group, 2001), 63.

3. Robert E. Buswell Jr. and Donald S. Lopez Jr., *The Princeton Dictionary of Buddhism,* (Princeton, NJ: Princeton University Press, 2014,), 817.

CHAPTER 1

1. Mohan Wijayaratna, *Buddhist Monastic Life*, (Cambridge: Cambridge University Press, 1990), 71.

2. Thanissaro Bhikkhu, *The Buddhist Monastic Code* (Valley Center, CA: Metta Forest Monastery, 1994), 362.

3. Wijayaratna, *Buddhist Monastic Life,* 181.

4. Bhikkhu Bodhi, *The Numerical Discourses of the Buddha* (Somerville, MA: Wisdom Publications, 2012), 1180.

5. Wijayaratna, *Buddhist Monastic Life*, 68.

6. Amandine Chaix et al. "Time-Restricted Feeding Is a Preventative and Therapeutic Intervention against Diverse Nutritional Challenges," *Cell Metabolism* 20, no. 6 (2014): 991–1005. doi:10.1016/j.cmet.2014.11.001.

7. Luigi Fontana and Frank B. Hu, "Optimal Body Weight for Health

and Longevity: Bridging Basic, Clinical, and Population Research."
Aging Cell 13, no. 3 (June 2014): 391–400. doi:10.1111/acel.12207.

8. Tapan Mehta, "Obesity and Mortality: Are the Risks Declining? Evidence from Multiple Prospective Studies in the U.S." *Obesity Review* 15, no. 8 (Aug. 2014): 619–29. doi:10.1111/12191.

9. Avi Dor, Christine Ferguson, Casey Langwith, and Ellen Tan. "A Heavy Burden: The Individual Costs of Being Overweight and Obese in the United States" (research report, The George Washington University, School of Public Health and Health Services, Department of Health Policy, Sep 21, 2010). http://hsrc.himmelfarb.gwu.edu/sphhs_policy_facpubs/212/.

10. Gallup News Service, "Gallup Poll Social Series: Health and Healthcare," November 7–10, 2013.

11. Bhikkhu Nanamoli and Bhikkhu Bodhi, *The Middle-Length Discourses of the Buddha* (Sommerville, MA: Wisdom Publications, 1995), 134.

CHAPTER 2

1. Walpola Rahula, *What the Buddha Taught* (New York, NY: Grove Press, 1974), 8.

2. Bhikku Bodhi, *In the Buddha's Words* (Sommerville, MA: Wisdom Publications, 1974), 98.

3. For example, in Marion Nestle's bestselling *What to Eat*: "When it comes to weight loss, it's the calories that count." But there are many, many examples. Marion Nestle, *What to Eat* (New York, NY: North Point Press, 2007), 283.

4. Gary Taubes cites many examples of studies showing the same thing: "Eating less—that is, undereating—simply doesn't work for more than a few months, if that." Gary Taubes, *Why We Get Fat* (New

York, NY: Anchor, 2011), 36.

5. Robert H. Lustig, *Fat Chance: Beating the Odds against Sugar, Processed Food, Obesity, and Disease* (New York, NY: Plume, 2013), 81.

6. Taubes, *Why We Get Fat*, 115.

7. Lustig, *Fat Chance*, 95–6.

8. Erica M. Schulte, Nicole M. Avena, Ashley N. Gearhardt, "Which Foods May Be Addictive? The Roles of Processing, Fat Content, and Glycemic Load," *PLoS ONE* 10, no. 2 (Feb. 18, 2015): e0117959. doi:10.1371/journal.pone.0117959.

9. Robert H. Lustig et al., "Isocaloric Fructose Restriction and Metabolic Improvement in Children with Obesity and Metabolic Syndrome," *Obesity* (Feb. 2015). doi:10.1002/oby.21371.

See, for example *The Sugar Detox* by Brooke Alpert and Patricia Farris, *Fat Chance* by Robert Lustig, and *Eat Bacon, Don't Jog* by Grant Petersen.

10. Mark P. Mattson et al., "Meal Frequency and Timing in Health and Disease," *PNAS* 111, no. 47 (November 25, 2014): 16648. doi:10.1073/pnas.1413965111.

11. Gary Taubes, *Good Calories, Bad Calories* (New York, NY: Anchor, 2008), 250.

CHAPTER 3

1. Steven W. Lichtman et al., "Discrepancy between Self-Reported and Actual Caloric Intake and Exercise in Obese Subjects," *New England Journal of Medicine* 327, no. 27 (Dec. 31, 1992): 1893–98. doi:10.1056/NEJM199212313272701.

2. Megan A. McCrory et al., "Eating Frequency and Energy Regulation in Free-Living Adults Consuming Self-Selected Diets," *Journal of Nutrition* 141, no. 27 (2011), 148–153. doi:10.3945/

jn.109.114991.

3. Sarah Shaw, trans., "The Story of the Hare," in *The Jātakas: Birth Stories of the Bodhisatta* (New York: Penguin Books, 2006), 114–121.

4. Thanissaro Bhikkhu, *Dhammapada: A Translation* (Valley Center, CA: Metta Forest Monastery, 2011), 67.

5. Megumi Hatori et al., "Time-Restricted Feeding without Reducing Caloric Intake Prevents Metabolic Diseases in Mice Fed a High-Fat Diet," *Cell Metabolism* 15, no. 6 (June 6, 2012): 848–60. doi:10.1016/j.cmet.2012.04.019.

6. Amandine Chaix et al., "Time-Restricted Feeding Is a Preventative and Therapeutic Intervention against Diverse Nutritional Challenges," *Cell Metabolism* 20, no. 6 (Dec. 2, 2014): 991–1005. doi:10.1016/j.cmet.2014.11.001.

7. James D. LeCheminant et al., "Restricting Night-Time Eating Reduces Daily Energy Intake in Healthy Young Men: A Short-Term Cross-Over Study," *British Journal of Nutrition* 110, no. 11 (Dec. 14, 2013): 2108–13. doi:10.1017/S0007114513001359.

8. Kim S. Stote et al., "A Controlled Trial of Reduced Meal Frequency without Caloric Restriction in Healthy, Normal-Weight, Middle-Aged Adults," *American Journal of Clinical Nutrition* 85, no. 4 (April 2007): 981–8.

9. Shubhroz Gill and Satchidananda Panda, "A Smartphone App Reveals Erratic Diurnal Eating Patterns in Humans that Can Be Modulated for Health Benefits," *Cell Metabolism* 22, no. 5 (Nov. 3, 2015): 789–798. doi:10.1016/j.cmet.2015.09.005.

CHAPTER 4

1. Gill and Panda, "Smartphone App," 1–10. (see chapter 3, n. 39).

2. Mark P. Mattson et al., "Meal Frequency and Timing in Health and Disease," *PNAS*, 111, no. 47 (Nov. 25, 2014): 16647. doi:10.1073/pnas.1413965111.

3. Daniela Jakubowicz et al., "High Caloric Intake at Breakfast vs. Dinner Differentially Influences Weight Loss of Overweight and Obese Women," *Obesity* 21, no. 12 (Dec. 2013): 2504–12. doi:10.1002/oby.20460.

4. Andrew W. McHill et al, "Impact of Circadian Misalignment on Energy Metabolism During Simulated Nightshift Work," *Proceedings of the National Academy of Science* 111, no. 48 (Dec. 2, 2014): vol. 7302–17307. doi:10.1073/pnas.1412021111.

5. Gill and Panda, "Smartphone App," 1–10. (see chap. 3, n. 39).

6. Grant Petersen, *Eat Bacon, Don't Jog.* (New York, NY: Workman Publishing, 2014), 7.

7. For example: Kim S. Stote et al., "Controlled Trial," 981–88. (see chap. 3, n. 8).

CHAPTER 5

1. Amanda M. Czerniawski, "From Average to Ideal: The Evolution of the Height and Weight Table in the United States, 1836–1943," *Social Science History* 31, no. 2 (Summer 2007): 273–296. doi:10.1215/01455532-2006-023.

2. Kate Crawford, Jessa Lingel, and Tero Karppi, "Our Metrics, Ourselves: A hundred Years of Self Tracking from the Weight Scale to the Wrist Wearable Device," *European Journal of Cultural Studies* 18, no. 4–5 (Aug.–Oct. 2015): 479–96. doi:10.1177/1367549415584857.

3. Yaguang Zheng et al., "Self-Weighing in Weight Management: A Systematic Literature Review," *Obesity* 23, no. 2 (Feb. 2015): 256–65. doi:10.1002/oby.20946.

4. Jeffrey J. VanWormer et al., "Self-Weighing Frequency Is Associated with Weight Gain Prevention over Two Years among Working Adults," *International Journal of Behavioral Medicine*. 19, no. 3 (September 2012): 351–58. doi:10.1007/s12529-011-9178-1.

5. Rena R. Wing et al., "A Self-Regulation Program for Maintenance of Weight Loss," *New England Journal of Medicine* 355, no. 15 (Oct. 12, 2006): 1563–71. doi:10.1056/NEJMoa061883.

6. Meghan L. Butryn et al., "Consistent Self-Monitoring of Weight: A Key Component of Successful Weight Loss Maintenance," *Obesity*. 15, no. 12 (December 2007): 3091. doi:10.1038/oby.2007.368.

7. Clément Rosset, *Loin de moi. Etude sur l'identité* (Paris, France: Editions de Minuit, 2001), 85–86.

CHAPTER 6

1. See Peter Menzel and Faith D'Aluisio, *What I Eat: Around the World in 80 Diets*, (Emeryville, CA: Ten Speed Press, 2010) for many examples.

2. Adam Drewnowski et al., "Sweetness and Food Preference," *Journal of Nutrition* 142, no. 6 (May 9, 2012): 1142S–48S. doi:10.3945/jn.111.149575.

3. Michael Moss, *Salt Sugar Fat*, (New York, NY: Random House, 2014), 10.

4. Julie A. Mennella et al., "Evaluation of the Monell Forced-Choice, Paired-Comparison Tracking Procedure for Determining Sweet Taste Preferences across the Lifespan," *Chemical Senses* 36, no. 4 (2011): 345–55. doi:10.1093/chemse/bjq134.

5. M. Yanina Pepino and Julie A. Mennella, "Habituation to the Pleasure Elicited by Sweetness in Lean and Obese Women," *Appetite*. 58, no. 3 (June 2012): 800–05. doi:10.1016/j.appet.2012.01.026.

6. Erica M. Schulte, Nicole M. Avena, and Ashley N. Gearhardt, "Which Foods May Be Addictive? The Roles of Processing, Fat Content, and Glycemic Load," *PLoS ONE* 10, no. 2 (February 18, 2015): e0117959. doi:10.1371/journal.pone.0117959.

7. Kevin J. Acheson et al., "Protein Choices Targeting Thermogenesis and Metabolism," *American Journal of Clinical Nutrition* 93, no. 3 (March 2011):525–34. doi:10.3945/ajcn.110.005850.

8. Abdou Himaya et al., "Satiety Power of Dietary Fat: a New Appraisal," *American Journal of Clinical Nutrition* 65, no. 5 (May 1997): 1410–18.

9. Joanne Harrold et al., "Satiety Effects of a Whole-Grain Fibre Composite Ingredient: Reduced Food Intake and Appetite Ratings," *Food & Function* 5, no. 10 (October 2014): 2574-2581. doi:10.1039/c4fo00253a.

10. Corinne Marmonier et al., "Snacks Consumed in a Nonhungry State Have Poor Satiating Fficiency: Influence of Snack Composition on Substrate Utilization and Hunger," *American Journal of Clinical Nutrition* 76, no. 3 (2002): 518–28.

11. CMarmonier et al./ "Snacks Consumed"

12. Marjet J. M. Munsters and Wim H. M. Saris, "Effects of Meal Frequency on Metabolic Profiles and Substrate Partitioning in Lean Healthy Males," *PLoS ONE* 7, no. 6 (June 13, 2012): e38632. doi:10.1371/journal.pone.0038632.

13. An Pana and Frank B. Hu, "Effects of Carbohydrates on Satiety: Differences Between Liquid and Solid Food," *Current Opinion in Clinical Nutrition and Metabolic Care* 14, no. 4 (July 2011):385–390. doi:10.1097/MCO.0b013e328346df36.

14. Ann V. Griffith et al., "Metabolic Damage and Premature Thymus Aging Caused by Stromal Catalase Deficiency," *Cell Reports* 12, no. 7 (August 18, 2015): 1071–1079. doi:10.1016/j.cel-

rep.2015.07.008.

15. Goran Bjelakovic et al., "Mortality in Randomized Trials of Antioxidant Supplements for Primary and Secondary Prevention: Systematic Review and Meta-analysis," *JAMA* 297, no. 8 (February 28, 2007): 842–857.

16. Jonathan D. Schoenfeld and John P.A. Ioannidis, "Is Everything We Eat Associated with Cancer? A Systematic Cookbook Review," *American Journal of Clinical Nutrition* 97, no. 1 (January 2013): 127–34. doi:10.3945/ajcn.112.047142.

17. Shubhroz Gill and Satchidananda Panda, "A Smartphone App Reveals Erratic Diurnal Eating Patterns in Humans that Can Be Modulated for Health Benefits," *Cell Metabolism* 22, no. 5 (Nov. 3, 2015): 789–798. doi:10.1016/j.cmet.2015.09.005.

18. David R. Just and Brian Wansink, "Fast Food, Soft Drink and Candy Intake Is Unrelated to Body Mass Index for 95% of American Adults," *Obesity Science & Practice* 1, no. 2 (2015): 126–130. doi:10.1002/osp4.14.

CHAPTER 7

1. D. Seyfort Ruegg, "Ahimsa and Vegetarianism in the History of Buddhism." *Buddhist Studies in Honour of Walpola Rahula* (London, UK: Gordon Fraser, 1980), 234–241.

2. Mohan Wijayaratna, *Buddhist Monastic Life* (Cambridge, UK: Cambridge University Press, 1990), 70.

3. Isaline Blew Horner, *The Book of Discipline*, vol. 1 (Melksham, Wilts, UK: Pali Text Society, 1938), 296–302.

4. Rajiv Chowdhury et al., "Association of Dietary, Circulating, and Supplement Fatty Acids With Coronary Risk: A Systematic Review and Meta-analysis," *Annals of Internal Medicine* 160, no. 6 (May 6,

2014): 398–406. doi:10.7326/M13-1788.

5. Timothy J Key, "Mortality in Vegetarians and Nonvegetarians: Detailed Findings from a Collaborative Analysis of 5 Prospective Studies," *American Journal of Clinical Nutrition* 70, no. 3 Suppl. (Sept 1999): 516S–24S.

6. "Position of the American Dietetic Association: Vegetarian Diets," *Journal of the American Dietetic Association* 109, no 7 (July 2009): 1266–1282.

7. Paul N. Appleby et al., "The Oxford Vegetarian Study: an Overview," *American Journal of Clinical Nutrition* 70, no. 3 Supply (Sept. 1999): 525S–31S.

8. Gary E. Fraser, "Associations Between Diet and Cancer, Ischemic Heart Disease, and All-Cause Mortality in Non-Hispanic White California Seventh-day Adventists," *American Journal of Clinical Nutrition* 70, no. 3 Supply (Sept. 1999): 532S–8S.

9. Yessenia Tantamango-Bartley et al., "Vegetarian Diets and the Incidence of Cancer in a Low-risk Population," *Cancer Epidemiology, Biomarkers, and Prevention* 22, no. 2 (February 2013): 286–94. doi:10.1158/1055-9965.EPI-12-1060; and Michael J. Orlich et al., "Vegetarian Dietary Patterns and the Risk of Colorectal Cancers," *JAMA Internal Medicine* 175, no. 5 (May 1, 2015): 767–776. doi:10.1001/jamainternmed.2015.59.

10. For example: Dagfinn Aune et al., "Red and Processed Meat Intake and Risk of Colorectal Adenomas: a Systematic Review and Meta-Analysis of Epidemiological Studies," *Cancer Causes & Control* 24, no. 4 (April 2013): 611–627.

11. "Position of the American Dietetic Association: Vegetarian Diets," *Journal of the American Dietetic Association* 109, no 7 (July 2009): 1266-1282.

12. Vernon R. Young and Peter L. Pellett, "Plant proteins in relation

to human protein and amino acid nutrition," *American Journal of Clinical Nutrition* 59, no. 5 Suppl. (May 1994): 1203S–l2S.

13. U.S. Department of Agriculture and U.S. Department of Health and Human Services. *Dietary Guidelines for Americans, 2010*, 7th Edition (Washington, DC: U.S. Government Printing Office, December 2010).

14. Sarah Shaw, *The Jātakas: Birth Stories of the Bodhisatta* (London, UK: Penguin Books, 2006).

15. Kari Hamershlag, *Meat Eater's Guide to Climate Change + Health* (Washington, DC: Environmental Working Group, 2012).

16. Frank Newport, "In U.S., 5% Consider Themselves Vegetarians," *Gallup* (July 26, 2012). http://www.gallup.com/file/poll/156224/Vegetarian_Vegan_120726.pdf.

17. Kari Hamershlag, *Meat Eater's Guide to Climate Change + Health* (Washington, DC: Environmental Working Group, 2012).

CHAPTER 8

1. Rupert Gethin, *Sayings of the Buddha: A selection of Suttas from the Pali Nikāyas* (Oxford, UK: Oxford University Press, 2008), 131.

2. Robert H. Lustig, *Fat Chance*, 122.

3. For example, Ilse C. Schrieks et al., "Moderate Alcohol Consumption Stimulates Food Intake and Food Reward of Savoury Foods," *Appetite* 89 (June 2015):77–83. doi:10.1016/j.appet.2015.01.021

4. Bhikkhu Bodhi, *The Numerical Discourse of the Buddha* (Somerville, MA: Wisdom Publications, 2012): 1176.

5. Robert H. Lustig, *Fat Chance,* 99.

6. Nina A.F.F. Furtwaengler and Richard O. de Visser, "Lack of International Consensus in Low-Risk Drinking Guidelines," *Drug and*

Alcohol Review 32, no. 1 (Jan. 2013): 11–18. doi:10.1111/j.1465-3362.2012.00475.x

7. K. Robertson et al., "Public Policy and Personal Preference: a Disconnect Between Beliefs Regarding Responsible Drinking and the Motivation to Get Drunk," *Public Health* 128, no. 11 (Nov. 2014): 1030–32. doi:10.1016/j.puhe.2014.08.006.

8. G. Galli et al, "Inverse Relationship of Food and Alcohol Intake to Sleep Measures in Obesity," *Nutrition and Diabetes* 3 (January 28, 2013): e58. doi:10.1038/nutd.2012.33.

9. Jongit Angkatvanich and Manee Zuesongdham, "Nutrition Problem Solving and Management Project for Monks and Novices," *International Buddhist Research Seminar* (Bangkok, Thailand: Buddhist Research Institute, Mahachulalongkornrajavidyalaya University, 2014), 1–7.

10. A. K. Lee, R. Chowdhury, and J. A. Welsh, "Sugars and Adiposity: the Long-Term Effects of Consuming Added and Naturally Occurring Sugars in Foods and in Beverages," *Obesity Science & Practice* 1, no.1 (October 2015), 41–49. doi:10.1002/osp4.7.

11. Geert Jan Biessels, "Caffeine, Diabetes, Cognition, and Dementia," *Journal of Alzheimer's Disease* 20, Suppl 1 (2010): S143–S150. doi:10.3233/JAD-2010-091228.

12. Marilyn C. Cornelis and Ahmed El-Sohemy, "Coffee, caffeine, and coronary heart disease," *Current Opinion in Lipidology* 18, no. 1 (February 2007): 13–19.

13. Uhee Lim, Patricia Hartge, Lindsay M. Morton, and Arthur Schatzkin. "Consumption of Aspartame-Containing Beverages and Incidence of Hematopoietic and Brain Malignancies," *Cancer Epidemiology, Biomarkers and Prevention* 15, no. 9 (Sept. 2006):1654–59.

14. Sara N. Bleich et al, "Diet-Beverage Consumption and Caloric

Intake Among US Adults, Overall and by Body Weight," *American Journal of Public Health*, March 2014, Vol. 104, No. 3, pp. 72-78.

15. Sharon P.G. Fowler et al., "Diet Soda Intake Is Associated With Long-Term Increases In Waist Circumference in a Bi-Ethnic Cohort of Older Adults: The San Antonio Longitudinal Study of Aging," *Journal of the American Geriatric Society* 63, no. 4(April 2015): 708–715. doi:10.1111/jgs.13376.

16. Jotham Suez et al., "Artificial Sweeteners Induce Glucose Intolerance by Altering the Gut Microbiota," *Nature* 514, no. 7521 (Oct. 9, 2014): 181–6. doi:10.1038/nature13793.

CHAPTER 9

1. Paul S. McLean et al., "Biology's Response to Dieting: the Impetus for Weight Regain," *American Journal of Physiology—Regulatory, Integrative and Comparative Physiology* 301, no 3 (September 2011): R581–R600. doi:10.1152/ajpregu.00755.2010.

2. Eric T. Trexler et al., "Metabolic Adaptation To Weight Loss: Implications For The Athlete," *Journal of the International Society of Sports Nutrition* 11, no 1 (Feb. 27, 2014): 7. doi:10.1186/1550-2783-11-7.

3. Leanne M. Redman et al., "Metabolic and Behavioral Compensations in Response to Caloric Restriction: Implications for the Maintenance of Weight Loss," *PLoS ONE* 4, no. 2 (2009): e4377. doi:10.1371/journal.pone.0004377.

4. Mirjam Dirlewanger et al., "Effects Of Short-Term Carbohydrate or Fat Overfeeding on Energy Expenditure and Plasma Leptin Concentrations in Healthy Female Subjects," *International Journal of Obesity Related Metabolic Disorders* 24, no. 11 (November 2000): 1413–8.

5. Todd A. Hagobian, Carrie G. Sharoff, and Barry Braun, "Effects of Short-Term Exercise and Energy Surplus on Hormones Related to Regulation of Energy Balance," *Metabolism* 57, no. 3 (March 2008):

393-8. doi:10.1016/j.metabol.2007.10.016

6. Eric T. Trexler et al., "Metabolic Adaptation to Weight Loss: Implications for the Athlete," *Journal of the International Society of Sports Nutrition* 11, no. 1 (Feb. 27, 2014): 7.

7. Rena R. Wing and Robert W. Jeffery, "Prescribed 'Breaks' as a Means to Disrupt Weight Control Efforts," *Obesity Research* 11, no. 2 (Feb. 2003): 287–291.

CHAPTER 10

1. Robert H. Lustig , *Fat Chance*, 50.

2. Gary Taubes, *Why We Get Fat*, 142–143.

3. Leandro Z. Agudelo et al., "Skeletal Muscle PGC-1⊠1 Modulates Kynurenine Metabolism and Mediates Resilience to Stress-Induced Depression." *Cell* 159, no. 1 (September 25, 2014): 33–45. doi:10.1016/j.cell.2014.07.051.

4. Thich Nhat Hanh, *The Long Road Turns to Joy: A Guide to Walking Meditation* (Berkeley, CA: Parallax Press, 2001), 7.

5. Steven Heine, *Dogen: Textual and Historical Studies* (Oxford, UK: Oxford University Press, 2012), 118.

6. Mark Mattson, personal communication, December 6, 2015.

7. Javier T. Gonzalez et al., "Breakfast and Exercise Contingently Affect Postprandial Metabolism and Energy Balance in Physically Active Males," *British Journal of Nutrition* 110, no. 4 (August 2013): 721–32. doi:10.1017/S0007114512005582.

8. Duck-chul Lee et al., "Leisure-Time Running Reduces All-Cause and Cardiovascular Mortality Risk," *Journal of the American College of Cardiology* 64, no. 5 (Aug. 5, 2014): 472–81. doi:10.1016/j.

jacc.2014.04.058.

9. Peter Schnohr et al., "Longevity in Male and Female Joggers: the Copenhagen City Heart Study," *American Journal of Epidemiology* 177, no. 7 (April 1, 2013): 683–689. doi:10.1093/aje/kws301

10. Philipe de Souto Barreto, "Global Health Agenda on Non-Communicable Diseases: Has WHO Set A Smart Goal for Physical Activity?" *British Medical Journal* 350 (Jan. 21, 2015: h23. doi:10.1136/bmj.h23.

11. Paul Carus, *The Gospel of Buddha* (Chicago, IL: The Open Court Publishing Company, 1894), 22.

CHAPTER 11

1. Bhikkhu Bodhi, *The Numerical Discourses of the Buddha: A Complete Translation of the Anguttara Nikaya* (Somerville, MA: Wisdom Publications, 2012), 933.

2. Maurice Walshe, *The Long Discourses of the Buddha: A Translation of the Digha Nikaya,* (Somerville, MA: Wisdom Publications, 1995), 463.

3. *Morbidity and Mortality Weekly Report* (Atlanta, GA: Centers for Disease Control and Prevention, March 4, 2011).

4. M. Garaulet et al., "The Chronobiology, Etiology and Pathophysiology of Obesity," *International Journal of Obesity (Lond).* 34, no. 12 (Dec. 2010): 1667-83. doi:10.1038/ijo.2010.118.

5. Guglielmo Beccuti, "Sleep and Obesity," *Current Opinion in Clinical Nutrition and Metabolic Care* 14, no. 4 (July 2011): 402–412. doi:10.1097/MCO.0b013e3283479109.

6. Jean-Philippe Chaput et al., "Do All Sedentary Activities Lead to Weight Gain: Sleep Does Not," *Current Opinion in Clinical Nutrition and Metabolic Care* 13, no. 6 (November 2010): 601–607.

doi:10.1097/MCO.0b013e32833ef30e.

7. Arlet V. Nedeltcheva et al., "Sleep Curtailment Is Accompanied by Increased Intake of Calories from Snacks," *American Journal of Clinical Nutrition* 89, no. 1 (Jan. 2009): 126–33. doi:10.3945/ ajcn.2008.26574.

8. Jean-Philippe Chaput and Angelo Tremblay, "Adequate Sleep to Improve the Treatment of Obesity," *Canadian Medical Association Journal* 184, no. 18 (Dec, 11, 2012): 1975–6. doi:10.1503/ cmaj.120876.

9. Julia S. Dweck, Steve M. Jenkins, and Laurence J. Nolan, "The Role of Emotional Eating and Stress in the Influence of Short Sleep on Food Consumption," *Appetite* 72 (Jan. 2014): 106–13. doi:10.1016/j.appet.2013.10.001.

10. Lisa L. Morselli et al., "Sleep and Metabolic Function," *Pflugers Archiv* 463, no. 1 (Jan. 2012): 139–160. doi:10.1007/s00424-011-1053-z.

11. Neomi Shah and Francoise Roux, "The Relationship of Obesity and Obstructive Sleep Apnea," *Clinics in Chest Medicine* 30, no. 3 (Sep. 2009): 455–465. doi:10.1016/j.ccm.2009.05.012.

12. Jean-Philippe Chaput and Angelo Tremblay, "Insufficient Sleep as a Contributor to Weight Gain: An Update," *Current Obesity Reports* 1, no. 4 (Dec. 2012): 245–256. doi:10.1007/s13679-012-0026-7.

13. M-L Filiatrault et al., "Eating Behavior Traits and Sleep as Determinants of Weight Loss in Overweight and Obese Adults," *Nutrition & Diabetes* 4 (2014): e140. doi:10.1038/nutd.2014.37.

14. Chaput and Tremblay, "Insufficient Sleep".

15. Charles R. Elder et al., "Impact of sleep, screen time, depression, and stress on weight change in the intensive weight loss phase of the LIFE study," *International Journal of Obesity* (London) 36, no. 1 (Jan. 2012): 86–92. doi:10.1038/ijo.2011.60.

16. Jean-Philippe and Chaputa Angelo Tremblay, "Sleeping Habits Predict the Magnitude of Fat Loss in Adults Exposed to Moderate Caloric Restriction," *Obesity Facts* 5, no. 4 (2012): 561–66. doi:10.1159/000342054.

17. Lundgren et al., "A Descriptive Study of Non-obese Persons with Night Eating Syndrome and a Weight-Matched Comparison Group," *Eating Behavior* 9, no. 3 (Aug. 2008): 343–351. doi:10.1016/j.eatbeh.2007.12.004. Also: Suat Kucukgoncu et al, "Optimal Management of Night Eating Syndrome: Challenges and Solutions," *Neuropsychiatric Disease and Treatment* 11 (Mar. 19, 2015): 751–760. doi:10.2147/NDT.S70312.

18. Bhikkhu Bodhi, *The Numerical Discourses of the Buddha: A Complete Translation of the Anguttara Nikaya*, (Somerville, MA: Wisdom Publications, 2012), 233.

19. Bhikkhu Nanamoli and Bhikkhu Bodhi, *The Middle Length Discourses of the Buddha: A Translation of the Majjhima Nikaya*, (Somerville, MA: Wisdom Publications, 1995), 1017.

20. T. Heidenreich et al., "Mindfulness-Based Cognitive Therapy for Persistent Insomnia: a Pilot Study," *Psychotherapy and Psychosomatics* 75, no. 3 (2006): 188–9.

21. Serge Brand et al., "The Relationship Between Physical Activity and Sleep From Mid Adolescence to Early Adulthood. A Systematic Review of Methodological Approaches and Meta-Analysis," *Sleep Medicine Review* 28 (Aug. 5, 2015): 28–41. doi:10.1016/j.smrv.2015.07.004.

22. For a whole book on this subject, see Joseph Emet, *Buddha's Book of Sleep* (New York, NY: Jeremy P. Tarcher, 2012).

23. Shawn D. Youngstedt and Christopher E. Kline, "Epidemiology of Exercise and Sleep," *Sleep and Biological Rhythms* 4, no. 3 (2006): 215–221.

24. Horacio O. de la Iglesia et al., "Access to Electric Light Is Associated with Shorter Sleep Duration in a Traditionally Hunter-Gatherer Community," *Journal of Biological Rhythms* 30, no. 4 (August 2015): 342–350. doi:10.1177/0748730415590702.

CHAPTER 12

1. Peggy Bongers et al., "Emotional Eating And Pavlovian Learning: Does Negative Mood Facilitate Appetitive Conditioning?" *Appetite* 89 (June 1, 2015): 226–236. doi:10.1016/j.appet.2015.02.018.

2. Michael Macht, Jutta Gerer, and Heiner Ellgring, "Emotions In Overweight and Normal-Weight Women Immediately After Eating Foods Differing in Energy," *Physiology & Behavior* 80, nos. 2–3 (Nov. 2003): 367–374. doi:10.1016/j.physbeh.2003.08.012.

3. Minati Singh, "Mood, Food, and Obesity," *Frontiers in Psychology* 5 (Sept. 1, 2014): 925. doi:10.3389/fpsyg.2014.00925.

4. Patricia Sue Grigson, "Like Drugs for Chocolate: Separate Rewards Modulated by Common Mechanisms?" *Physiology & Behavior* 76, no. 3 (2002): 389–395.

5. Lukas Van Oudenhove et al., "Fatty Acid–Induced Gut-Brain Signaling Attenuates Neural and Behavioral Effects of Sad Emotion in Humans," *Journal of Clinical Investigation* 121, no. 8 (Aug. 2011): 3094–99. doi:10.1172/JCI46380.

6. Edward Leigh Gibson, "Emotional Influences on Food Choice: Sensory, Physiological and Psychological Pathways," *Physiology & Behavior* 89, no. 1 (Aug. 30, 2006): 53–61.

7. Janice K. Kiecolt-Glaser et al., "Daily Stressors, Past Depression, and Metabolic Responses to High-Fat Meals: a Novel Path to Obesity," *Biological Psychiatry* 77, no. 7 (Apr. 1, 2015): 653-60. doi:10.1016/j.biopsych.2014.05.018.

8. Michael Macht, Jutta Gerer, and Heiner Ellgring, "Emotions In Overweight and Normal-Weight Women Immediately After Eating Foods Differing in Energy," *Physiology & Behavior* 80, nos. 2–3 (Nov. 2003): 367–374. doi:10.1016/j.physbeh.2003.08.012.

9. Minati Singh, "Mood, Food, and Obesity," *Frontiers in Psychology* 5 (Sept. 1, 2014): 925. doi:10.3389/fpsyg.2014.00925.

10. Sonja T.P. Spoora et al., "Relations Between Negative Affect, Coping, and Emotional Eating," *Appetite* 48, no. 3 (2007): 368–76. doi:10.1016/j.appet.2006.10.005.

11. Normal S. Endler and James D. A. Parker, "Multidimensional Assessment of Coping: a Critical Evaluation," *Journal of Social and Personality Psychology*, 58, no. 5 (May 1990): 844–54. doi:10.1037/0022-3514.58.5.844.

12. Amber W. Li and Carroll-Ann W. Goldsmith, "The Effects of Yoga on Anxiety and Stress," *Alternative Medicine Review* 17, no. 1. (2012): 21–35.

13. Deborah R. Simkin and Nancy B. Black, "Meditation and Mindfulness in Clinical Practice," *Child and Adolescent Psychiatric Clinics of North America* 23, no. 3 (July 2014): 487–534. doi:10.1016/j.chc.2014.03.002.

14. Kaushadh Jayakody, Shalmini Gunadasa, and Christian Hosker, "Exercise for Anxiety Disorders: Systematic Review," *British Journal of Sports Medicine* 48, no. 3 (Feb 2014): 187–96. doi:10.1136/bjsports-2012-091287.

15. Rita Berto, "The Role of Nature in Coping with Psycho-Physiological Stress: A Literature Review on Restorativeness," *Behavioral Science (Basel)* 4, no 4 (Oct. 21, 2014): 394–409. doi:10.3390/bs4040394.

16. Rebecca M. Puhl and Marlene B. Schwartz, "If You Are Good You Can Have a Cookie: How Memories of Childhood Food Rules Link to Adult Eating Behaviors," *Eating Behaviors* 4, no. 3 (Sept.

2003): 283–93. doi:10.1016/S1471-0153(03)00024-2.

17. Laurel Branen and Janice Fletcher, "Comparison of College Students' Current Eating Habits and Recollections of Their Childhood Food Practices," *Journal of Nutrition Education* 31, no. 6 (Nov. 1999): 304–10. doi:10.1016/S0022-3182(99)70483-8.

18. Edward Leigh Gibson, "Emotional Influences on Food Choice: Sensory, Physiological and Psychological Pathways," *Physiology & Behavior* 89, no. 1 (Aug. 30, 2006): 53–61. doi:10.1016/j.physbeh.2006.01.024.

19. Michael Macht, Jutta Gerer, and Heiner Ellgring, "Emotions In Overweight and Normal-Weight Women Immediately After Eating Foods Differing in Energy," *Physiology & Behavior* 80, nos. 2–3 (Nov. 2003): 367–74. doi:10.1016/j.physbeh.2003.08.012.

20. Uma R. Karmarkar and Bryan Bollinger (2015) "BYOB: How Bringing Your Own Shopping Bags Leads to Treating Yourself and the Environment," *Journal of Marketing* 79, no. 4 (July 2015): 1–15. doi:10.1509/jm.13.0228.

CHAPTER 13

1. Thanaissaro Bhikkhi, *The Buddhist Monastic Code* (Valley Center, CA: Metta Forest Monastery, 2013): 497.

2. See, for example: Susan Albers, *Eating Mindfully* (Oakland, CA: New Harbinger Publications, 2012).

3. Brian Wansink and Jeffery Sobal, "Mindless Eating: The 200 Daily Food Decisions We Overlook," *Environment and Behavior* 39, no. 1 (Jan. 2007): 106–23. doi:10.1177/0013916506295573.

4. Brian Wansink and Junyong Kim, "Bad Popcorn in Big Buckets: Portion Size Can Influence Intake as Much as Taste," *Journal of Nutrition Education and Behavior* 37, no. 5 (Sept. – Oct. 2005): 242–5.

[5] Kirsikka Kaipainen, Collin R Payne, and Brian Wansink, "Mindless Eating Challenge: Retention, Weight Outcomes, and Barriers for Changes in a Public Web-Based Healthy Eating and Weight Loss Program," *Journal of Medical Internet Research* 14, no. 6 (Dec. 17, 2012): e168. doi:10.2196/jmir.2218.

[6] Lisa M. Jaremka et al., "Novel Links Between Troubled Marriages and Appetite Regulation: Marital Distress, Ghrelin, and Diet Quality," *Clinical Psychological Science* (July 29, 2015): 2167702615593714. doi:10.1177/2167702615593714.

[7] Robert Lustig, *Fat Chance*, 39.

[8] Wansink and Sobal, "Mindless Eating."

[9] Brian Wansink, James E. Painter, and Jill North, "Bottomless Bowls: Why Visual Cues of Portion Size May Influence Intake," *Obesity Research* 13, no. 1 (Jan. 2005):93–100.

CHAPTER 14

[1] Lisa M. Jaremka et al., "Interpersonal Stressors Predict Ghrelin and Leptin Levels in Women," *Psychoneuroendocrinology* 48, (Oct. 2014): 178–88. doi:10.1016/j.psyneuen.2014.06.018.

[2] Silvia Scaglioni et al., "Influence Of Parental Attitudes in the Development of Children Eating Behaviour," *British Journal of Nutrition* 99, Suppl. 1 (Feb. 2008): S22–S25. doi:10.1017/S0007114508892471.

[3] Rachel Brown and Jane Ogden, "Children's Eating Attitudes and Behaviour: a Study of the Modelling and Control Theories of Parental Influence," *Health Education Research* 19, no.3 (June 2004): 261–71. doi:10.1093/her/cyg040.

[4] Emma Dickens and Jane Ogden, "The Role of Parental Control and Modelling in Predicting a Child's Diet and Relationship with Food

After They Leave Home. a Prospective Study," *Appetite* 76 (May 2014) 23–29. doi:10.1016/j.appet.2014.01.013

5. Dickens and Ogden, "The Role of Parental Control".

6. Marla E. Eisenberg et al, "Associations Between Hurtful Weight-Related Comments by Family and Significant Other and the Development of Disordered Eating Behaviors in Young Adults," *Journal of Behavioral Medicine* 35, no. 5 (Oct. 2012): 500–8. doi:10.1007/s10865-011-9378-9.

7. Marla E. Eisenberg et al., "Dieting and encouragement to diet by significant others: associations with disordered eating in young adults," *American Journal of Health Promotion* 27, no. 6 (July–Aug. 2013): 370–377. doi:10.4278/ajhp.120120-QUAN-57.

8. Lisa M. Jaremka et al., "Novel Links Between Troubled Marriages and Appetite Regulation: Marital Distress, Ghrelin, and Diet Quality," *Clinical Psychological Science* (July 29, 2015): 2167702615593714. doi:10.1177/2167702615593714.

CHAPTER 15

1. John P. Trougakos et al., "Lunch Breaks Unpacked: The Role of Autonomy as a Moderator of Recovery during Lunch," *Academy of Management Journal* 57, no. 2 (Apr. 2014): 405–21. doi:10.5465/amj.2011.1072.

2. Jessica de Bloom, Ulla Kinnunen, and Kalevi Korpela, "Exposure To Nature Versus Relaxation During Lunch Breaks And Recovery From Work: Development And Design Of An Intervention Study To Improve Workers' Health, Well-Being, Work Performance And Creativity," *BMC Public Health* 14, (May 22, 2014): 488. doi:10.1186/1471-2458-14-488.

3. John P. Trougakos et al., "Lunch Breaks Unpacked: The Role of Autonomy as a Moderator of Recovery during Lunch," *Academy of Management Journal* 57, no. 2 (Apr. 2014): 405–21. doi:10.5465/

amj.2011.1072.

4. Jerica M. Berge, Nicole Larson, Katherine W. Bauer and Dianne Neumark-Sztainer, "Are Parents of Young Children Practicing Healthy Nutrition and Physical Activity Behaviors?" *Pediatrics* 127, no. 5 (May 2011): 881–7. doi:10.1542/peds.2010-3218.

5. Erik Dane, "Paying Attention to Mindfulness and Its Effects on Task Performance in the Workplace," *Journal of Management* 37, no. 4 (July 2011): 997-1018. doi:10.1177/0149206310367948.

6. Erik Dane and Bradley J Brummel, "Examining workplace mindfulness and its relations to job performance and turnover intention," *Human Relations* 67 (2014): 105–128. doi:10.1177/0018726713487753.

7. R. S. Kudesia, "Mindfulness and Creativity in the Workplace," in J. Reb and P. W. B. Atkins (eds.) *Mindfulness in Organisations* (Cambridge: Cambridge University Press, 2015).

8. C. Thøgersen-Ntoumani et al., "Changes In Work Affect In Response To Lunchtime Walking In Previously Physically Inactive Employees: A Randomized Trial," *Scandinavian Journal of Medicine & Science in Sports* 25, no. 6 (Dec. 2015): 778–87. doi:10.1111/sms.12398.

9. Peter Aspinall et al., "The Urban Brain: Analysing Outdoor Physical Activity with Mobile EEG," *British Journal of Sports Medicine,* 49, no. 4 (Feb. 2015): 272–76. doi:10.1136/bjsports-2012-091877.

10. Reza Amani and Tim Gill, "Shiftworking, Nutrition and Obesity: Implications for Workforce Health: a Systematic Review," *Asia Pacific Journal of Clinical Nutrition* 22, no. 4 (2013): 505-15. doi:10.6133/apjcn.2013.22.4.11.

11. Jonathan D. Johnston, "Physiological Responses to Food Intake Throughout the Day," *Nutrition Research Reviews* 27, no. 1 (June 2014): 107–118. doi:10.1017/S0954422414000055.

12. Stephen B. Hanauer, "Jet Lag: Life in the Fast (and Feast) Lane,"

Nature Clinical Practice Gastroenterology & Hepatology 5, no. 7 (2008): 349. doi:10.1038/ncpgasthep1187.

13. Till Roenneberg et al., "Social Jetlag and Obesity," *Current Biology* 22, no. 10 (May 22, 2012), 939–43. doi:10.1016/j. cub.2012.03.038.

14. Patricia M. Wong et al, "Social Jetlag, Chronotype, and Cardiometabolic Risk," *The Journal of Clinical Endocrinology & Metabolism* 100, no. 12 (November 18, 2015) :4612–20. doi:10.1210/jc.2015-2923

CHAPTER 16

1. Brian Lipinski et al., "Reducing Food Loss and Waste," Working Paper, Installment 2 of *Creating a Sustainable Food Future*. (Washington, DC: World Resources Institute, June 2013). http://www. worldresourcesreport.org.

2. Brian Lipinski et al., "Reducing Food Loss and Waste".

3. Rebecca M. Puhl and Marlene B. Schwartz, "If You Are Good You Can Have a Cookie: How Memories of Childhood Food Rules Link to Adult Eating Behaviors," *Eating Behaviors* 4, no. 3 (Sept. 2003): 283–93. doi:10.1016/S1471-0153(03)00024-2.

4. Norms and Win-Win Solutions for Reducing Food Intake and Waste," *Journal of Experimental Psychology: Applied* 19, no. 4, (Dec. 2013): 320–332. doi:10.1037/a0035053.

5. Koert van Ittersum and Brian Wansink, "Plate Size and Color Suggestibility: The Delboeuf Illusion's Bias on Serving and Eating Behavior," *Journal of Consumer Research* 39, no. 2 (August 2012): 215–28. doi:10.1086/662615.

6. B. Wansink and C.S. Wansink, "The Largest Last Supper: Depictions of Food Portions and Plate Size Increased Over the Millenni-

um," *International Journal of Obesity* 34, no. 5 (May 2010): 943–44. doi:10.1038/ijo.2010.37.

7. Koert van Ittersum and Brian Wansink, "Plate Size and Color Suggestibility: The Delboeuf Illusion's Bias on Serving and Eating Behavior," *Journal of Consumer Research* 39, no. 2 (August 2012): 215–28. doi:10.1086/662615.

8. Mary Kay Fox et al, "Relationship between Portion Size and Energy Intake among Infants and Toddlers: Evidence of Self-Regulation," *Journal of the American Dietetic Association* 106, no. 1, Suppl. (Jan. 2006): S77-83. doi:10.1016/j.jada.2005.09.039.

9. Leann L. Birch, Jennifer Orlet Fisher, and Kirsten Krahnstoever Davison, "Learning to Overeat: Maternal Use of Restrictive Feeding Practices Promotes Girls' Eating in the Absence Of Hunger," *American Journal of Clinical Nutrition* 78, no. 2 (Aug. 2003): 215–20.

10. T.E. Quested et al., "Spaghetti Soup: the Complex World of Food Waste Behaviours," *Resources, Conservation and Recycling* 79 (Oct. 2013): 43–51. doi:10.1016/j.resconrec.2013.04.011.

11. Alexandra Betz et al., "Food Waste in the Swiss Food Service Industry—Magnitude and Potential for Reduction," *Waste Management* 35 (Jan. 2015): 218–226. doi:10.1016/j.wasman.2014.09.015.

CHAPTER 17

1. Charles Duhigg, *The Power of Habit*, (New York, NY: Random House, 2012).

2. Charles Duhigg, *The Power of Habit*, 19.

3. Benjamin Gardner and Gert-Jan de Bruijn, "A Systematic Review and Meta-analysis of Applications of the Self-Report Habit Index to Nutrition and Physical Activity Behaviours," *Annals of Behavioral*

Medicine 42, no. 2 (Oct. 2011): 174–187. doi:10.1007/s12160-011-9282-0

4. Charles Duhigg, *The Power of Habit*, 78.

5. John B. Arden, *Rewire Your Brain* (New York, NY: John Wiley & Sons, 2010), 19.

6. Alan R. Andreasen, "Life Status Changes and Changes in Consumer Preferences and Satisfaction," *Journal of Consumer Research* 11, no. 3 (Dec. 1984): 784–94. doi:10.1086/209014.

7. Anil Mathur, George P. Moschis, and Euehun Lee, "A Longitudinal Study Of The Effects Of Life Status Changes On Changes In Consumer Preferences," *Journal of the Academy of Marketing Science* 36, no. 2 (May 2008): 234–246. doi:10.1007/s11747-007-0021-9.

CHAPTER 18

1. J.L. Kraschnewski, "Long-Term Weight Loss Maintenance in the United States," *International Journal of Obesity (London)* 34, no. 11 (Nov. 2010): 1644–54. doi:10.1038/ijo.2010.94.

2. Mary L. Kiem, "A Descriptive Study of Individuals Successful at Long-Term Maintenance of Substantial Weight Loss," *American Journal of Clinical Nutrition* 66, no. 2 (Aug. 1997): 239–46.

3. Paul S. MacLean et al, "Biology's response to dieting: the impetus for weight regain," *American Journal of Physiology—Regulatory, Integrative and Comparative Physiology*, 301, no. 3 (Sept. 2011): R581–R600. doi:10.1152/ajpregu.00755.2010.

4. Jeffrey J. VanWormer et al., "Self-weighing Frequency is Associated with Weight Gain Prevention over Two Years among Working Adults," *International Journal of Behavioral Medicine* 19, no. 3 (Sept. 2012): 351–58. doi:10.1007/s12529-011-9178-1.

5. Rena R. Wing and Suzanne Phelan, "Long-Term Weight Loss Main-

tenance," *American Journal of Clinical Nutrition* 82, no. 1, Suppl. (July 2005): 222S–5S.

6. Lucienne Roh, "Mortality Risk Associated with Underweight: a Census-Linked Cohort of 31,578 Individuals with up to 32 Years of Follow-up," *BMC Public Health* 14, (Apr. 16, 2014): 371. doi:10.1186/1471-2458-14-371

CHAPTER 19

1. Lacey Arneson et al., "Review of the Nutritional Implications of Farmers' Markets and Community Gardens: A Call for Evaluation and Research Efforts," *Journal of the American Dietetic Association* 110, no. 3 (Mar. 2010): 399-408. doi:10.1016/j.jada.2009.11.023.

2. Ramona Robinson-O'Brien et al., "Impact of Garden-Based Youth Nutrition Intervention Programs: A Review," *Journal of the American Dietetic Association* 109, no. 2 (Feb. 2009): 273–80. doi:10.1016/j.jada.2008.10.051.

3. Harold G. Koenig, "Religion, Spirituality, and Health: The Research and Clinical Implications," *International Scholarly Research Network ISRN Psychiatry* 2012 (Dec. 16. 2012): 278730. doi:10.5402/2012/278730.

4. Napaporn Sowattanangoon, Naipinich Kochabhakdi, and Keith J. Petrie, "Buddhist Values Are Associated with Better Diabetes Control in Thai Patients," *International Journal of Psychiatry Medicine* 38, no. 4 (2008): 481–91. doi:10.2190/PM.38.4.g.

5. Leslie A. Lytle et al., "Predicting Adolescents' Intake of Fruits and Vegetables," *Journal of Nutrition Education and Behavior* 35, no. 4 (June 2003): 170–5.

6. Bhikkhu Bodhi, *The Middle Length Discourses of the Buddha*, (Somerville, MA: Wisdom Publications, 2009), 811.

7. Wilhelm Hofmann et al., "Morality in Everyday Life," *Science* 345, no. 6202 (Sept. 12, 2014): 1340-1343. doi:10.1126/science.1251560.

8. Jean Decety et al, "The Negative Association between Religiousness and Children's Altruism across the World," *Current Biology* 25, no. 22 (Nov. 16, 2014): 2951–5. doi:10.1016/j.cub.2015.09.056.

CHAPTER 20

1. Maria Kozhevnikov, James Elliott, Jennifer Shephard, and Klaus Gramann, "Neurocognitive and Somatic Components of Temperature Increases during g-Tummo Meditation: Legend and Reality," *PLoS ONE* 8, no. 3 (Mar. 29, 2013): e58244. doi:10.1371/journal.pone.0058244.

2. Karen Armstrong, *Buddha* (New York, NY: Penguin Putnam, 2001), 80.

3. Bhikkhu Nanamoli and Bhikkhu Bodhi, *The Middle Length Discourses of the Buddha,* 155.

4. Bhikkhu Nanamoli and Bhikkhu Bodhi, *The Middle Length Discourses of the Buddha,* 145.

5. Julien Lacaille, at el., "The Effects of Three Mindfulness Skills on Chocolate Cravings," *Appetite* 76 (May 2014): 101–12. doi:10.1016/j.appet.2014.01.072.

6. H.J.E.M. Alberts, R. Thewissen, and L. Raes, "Dealing with Problematic Eating Behaviour: the Effects of a Mindfulness-Based Intervention on Eating Behaviour, Food Cravings, Dichotomous Thinking and Body Image Concern," *Appetite* 58, no. 3 (June 2012): 847-51. doi:10.1016/j.appet.2012.01.009.

7. Gillian A. O'Reilly et al., "Mindfulness-Based Interventions for Obesity-Related Eating Behaviors: A Literature Review," *Obesity Review* 15, no. 6 (June 2014): 453–61. doi:10.1111/obr.12156.

8. KayLoni L. Olson and Charles F. Emery, "Mindfulness and Weight Loss: A Systematic Review," *Psychosomatic Medicine* 77, no. 1 (Jan. 2015), 59–67. doi:10.1097/PSY.0000000000000127.

9. Shian-Ling Keng, Moria J. Smoski, and Clive J. Robins, "Effects of Mindfulness on Psychological Health: A Review of Empirical Studies," *Clinical Psychology Review,* 31, no. 6 (Aug. 2011): 1041–56. doi:10.1016/j.cpr.2011.04.006 .

10. Bhikkhu Nanamoli and Bhikkhu Bodhi, *The Middle Length Discourses of the Buddha,* 145.

11. See, for example, James H. Austin, *Zen and the Brain,* (Cambridge, MA: The MIT Press, 1999).

12. Yi-Yuan Tang, Britta K. Hölzel, and Michael I. Posner, "The neuroscience of mindfulness meditation," *Nature Reviews of Neuroscience* 16, no. 4 (April 2015): 213-25. doi:10.1038/nrn3916

13. Stephen Batchelor, *Buddhism Without Beliefs,* (New York, NY: Riverhead Books, 1997). 62–63.

14. Bhikkhu Nanamoli and Bhikkhu Bodhi, *The Middle Length Discourses of the Buddha,*146.

15. Joaquim Soler et al., "Relationship between Meditative Practice and Self-Reported Mindfulness: The MINDSENS Composite Index," *PLoS ONE* 9, no. 1 (Jan. 22, 2014): e86622. doi:10.1371/ journal.pone.0086622.

CHAPTER 21

1. Bhikkhu Bodhi, *The Connected Discourses of the Buddha* (Somerville, MA: Wisdom Publications, 2000), 1737.

2. Benjamin Gardner, Gert-Jan de Bruijn, and Phillippa Lally, "A Systematic Review and Meta-analysis of Applications of the Self-Report Habit Index to Nutrition and Physical Activity Behaviours," Annals

of Behavioral Medicine 42, no. 2 (Oct. 2011):174–87. doi:10.1007/
s12160-011-9282-0.

3. Trisha A. Pruis and Jeri S. Janowsky (2010) "Assessment of Body
Image in Younger and Older Women," *The Journal of General Psychology* 137, no. 3 (July–Sept. 2010): 225-238. doi:10.1080/00221
309.2010.484446.

4. Stephanie R. Damiano et al., "Relationships Between Body Size Attitudes and Body Image of 4-Year-Old Boys and Girls, and Attitudes
of Their Fathers and Mothers," *Journal of Eating Disorders* 3 (Apr.
10, 2015): 16. doi:10.1186/s40337-015-0048-0.

5. Nadia Micali et al., "Frequency and Patterns of Eating Disorder
Symptoms in Early Adolescence," *Journal of Adolescent Health* 54,
no. 5 (May 2014): 574–81. doi:10.1016/j.jadohealth.2013.10.200.

6. A. Janet Tomiyama and Traci Mann, "If Shaming Reduced Obesity,
There Would Be No Fat People," *The Hastings Center Report* 43, no.
3 (May–June 2013): 4–5. doi:10.1002/hast.166.

7. Angelina R. Sutin and Antonio Terracciano, "Perceived Weight
Discrimination and Obesity," *PLoS ONE* 8, no. 7(July 24, 2013):
e70048. doi:10.1371/journal.pone.0070048.

8. Gary D. Foster, Thomas A. Wadden, and Renee A. Vogt, "Body
Image in Obese Women Before, During, and After Weight Loss
Treatment," *Health Psychology* 16, no.3 (May 1997): 226–29.
doi:10.1037/0278-6133.16.3.226.

9. James J. Annesi and Nicole Mareno, "Improvement in Emotional
Eating Associated with an Enhanced Body Image in Obese Women:
Mediation by Weight-Management Treatments' Effects on Self-Ef-
ficacy To Resist Emotional Cues to Eating," *Journal of Advances in
Nursing* 71, no. 12 (Dec. 2015): 2923–35. doi:10.1111/jan.12766.

10. Hai-Lun Chao, "Body Image Change in Obese and Overweight
Persons Enrolled in Weight Loss Intervention Programs: A Sys-

tematic Review and Meta-Analysis," *PLoS ONE* 10, no. 5 (May 6, 2015): e0124036. doi:10.1371/journal.pone.0124036.

11. Kazuaki Tanahashi, *Treasury of the True Dharma Eye: Zen Master Dogen's Shobo Genzo* (Boulder, CO: Shambhala Publications, 2013), 347.

CHAPTER 22

1. Bhikkhu Bodhi, "What Does Mindfulness Really Mean? A Canonical Perspective," *Contemporary Buddhism*, 12, no. 1 (May 2011): 19–39. doi:10.1080/14639947.2011.564813.

2. Andrew Olendzki, "The Mindfulness Wedge," *Tricycle*, Fall 2014.

3. Lynette M. Monteiro, R.F. Musten, and Jane Compson, "Traditional And Contemporary Mindfulness: Finding The Middle Path In The Tangle Of Concerns," *Mindfulness* 6, no. 1 (Feb. 2015): 1–13. doi:10.1007/s12671-014-0301-7.

4. Bhikkhu Bodhi, *The Connected Discourses of the Buddha* (Somerville, MA: Wisdom Publications, 2000), 1844.

5. Robert Gethin, "On Some Definitions of Mindfulness," *Contemporary Buddhism* 12, no. 1 (May 2011): 263–79. doi:10.108 0/14639947.2011.564843.

6. Bhikkhu Nanamoli and Bhikkhu Bodhi, *The Middle Length Discourses of the Buddha* (Somerville, MA: Wisdom Publications, 1995), 301.

7. William L. Mikulas, "Ethics in Buddhist Training," *Mindfulness* 6, no. 1 (Feb. 2015): 14–16. doi:10.1007/s12671-014-0371-6.

8. Gill Fronsdal (trans.), *The Dhammapada* (Boulder, CO: Shambhala Publications, 2006), 1.

9. The Dalai Lama, *Kindness, Clarity, and Insight* (Ithaca, NY: Snow Lion Publications, 1984), 35.

10. Maurice Walshe, *The Long Discourses of the Buddha* (Somerville,

MA: Wisdom Publications, 1987), 397–398.

11. Marcia Keegan (ed.), *Teachings of His Holiness the Dalai Lama: The Dalai Lama's Historic Visit to North America* (New York, NY: Clear Light Publications, 1981), n. pag.

12. Bhikkhu Bodhi, *The Connected Discourses of the Buddha* (Somerville, MA, Wisdom Publications, 2000), 1264.

13. Kazuaki Tanahashi (ed.), *Moon in a Dewdrop: Writing of Zen Master Dōgen* (New York, NY: North Point Press, 1985), 70.

CHAPTER 23

1. Robert E. Buswell Jr. and Donald S. Lopez Jr., *The Princeton Dictionary of Buddhism* (Princeton, NJ: Princeton University Press, 2014), 693.

index

fruit juices, 84
guidelines for, 69–70
nonalcoholic drinks, 84–87
sodas, 84, 86
tea, 67, 85, 87
water, 84–85
whiskey, 83
wine, 81–83
Duhigg, Charles, 152, 153

E

Eating guidelines
for 9-hour window, 54–57
for 10-hour window, 52–54
for 11-hour window, 50–52
for 12-hour window, 48–50
exercise and, 97–98
meal schedules, 23–27, 38–40,
44–45, 126–132
for meals, 69–72
for snacks, 69–72
untimely eating and, 23–24, 27,
46–47
Eating habits, changing, 48–50,
56–57, 150–157
Eating round-the-clock, 46–47, 138,
155
Eightfold Path, 189–190
Einstein, Albert, 100
Eleven-hour window, 50–52
Emotional Eating, 114–115, 122. See
also Overeating
Enlightenment
achieving, 17–18, 173–175, 180–181,
188
explanation of, 174–175
meditation for, 173–175, 180–181
"Evil actions," 103–104

Exercise
benefits of, 94–96, 159–160
burning calories, 94–95, 98
diet and, 94–95
before eating, 97–98
jogging, 98–99
running, 94, 98–99
sleep and, 105
walking, 96–99, 137–138
weight loss and, 94–95, 159–160

F

Fad diets, 19, 70–71, 158–159
Family meals, 128–132
Fat
cholesterol and, 19
insulin and, 32–33
properties of, 69
saturated fat, 75, 136
sugar and, 19, 32–33, 66
weight gain and, 32–33, 66
Fiber, 69, 72, 156
Food
addictive foods, 35, 66–68, 95–96,
112–115
changing views on, 19
chewing, 119, 123–124
comfort foods, 110–114, 122
energy from, 31–32
importance of, 17, 29–32, 66
junk food, 49, 71–72, 117, 120, 153,
187
meal schedules, 23–27, 38–40,
44–45, 126–132
metabolism of, 31–32
overeating, 31–33, 86, 90–92,
114–115, 122–124, 128, 142–149
portion sizes, 145–146, 149–151

About the Authors

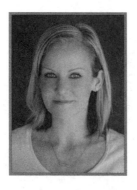

Tara Cottrell is a writer, digital strategist, and mom. She consults and writes for lifestyle and wellness brands in Silicon Valley and is an advocate for at-risk youth. She is currently the web content manager at Stanford University's Graduate School of Business. When she's not working, writing, or parenting, she's shoe shopping. She lives in Palo Alto, CA.

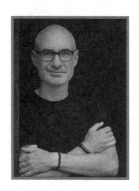

Dan Zigmond is a writer, data scientist, and Zen priest. He is Director of Analytics at Facebook, and advises start-ups and venture capital firms about data and health. He is a contributing editor at *Tricycle*, the largest Buddhist magazine in North America, and teaches at Jikoji Zen Center, a small Buddhist temple in the Santa Cruz mountains. In May 2015, he was named one of "20 Business Geniuses You Need to Know" by *Wired* magazine, as he frequently reminds his kids. He lives in Menlo Park, CA.